Take that...
and take *THAT!*

Twenty-Eight Years Surviving Parkinson's Disease ... and Still Counting

Martha Kowal

Sing the song that only you can sing,
write the book that only you can write,
build the product that only you can build . . .
live the life that only you can live.
—Naval Ravikant

Dedication

For my dear cousin Sally Donavon Goodrich, and for Marcia Gibbons, my good friend from Kittery. Both of these beautiful women died much too early of ovarian cancer. Both showed us how to live life to the fullest.

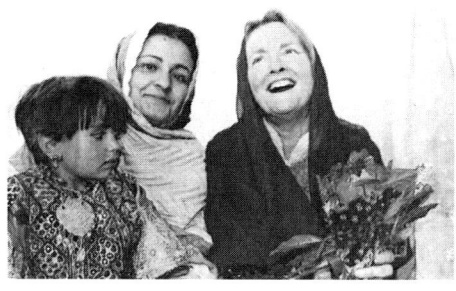

Sally, with her husband Don Goodrich, founded the Peter M. Goodrich Foundation in honor of their son Peter who was killed on 9-11. With funds raised in Peter's memory they dealt with their grief by courageously building a school in Afghanistan for five hundred girls. Sally traveled several times to Afghanistan, sometimes by herself, putting her life in danger. She was selfless, caring, determined, compassionate and fun to be with. She lovingly called me "Cuz."

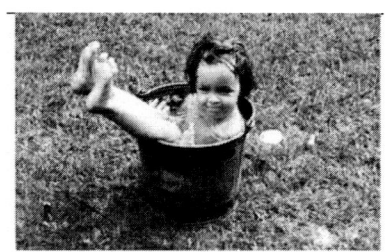

Sally getting off to a good start.

Marcia Gibbons was a locally known artist with many of her paintings hanging in our homes. She was a gardener extraordinaire and an incredibly remarkable woman. She always thought 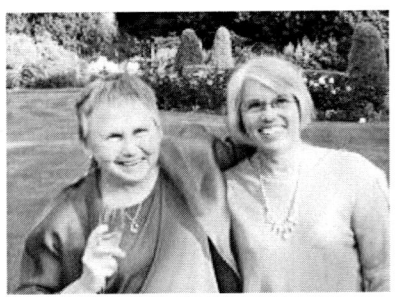 *of others. She acted as my cheerleader in my moving to Kittery Point. Once here, Marcia took me under her wing and introduced me to lots of people both from the church and the community.*

Both Sally and Marcia taught me to be positive in the face of adversity, to value friendships and family, to love always, to laugh and have a good time.

With Great Thanks

This memoir could not have happened without the support of Tessa Melvin, who has been an especially good friend for more than sixty years. She has always been honest and direct with me. Tessa guided me through the entire process of writing this book.

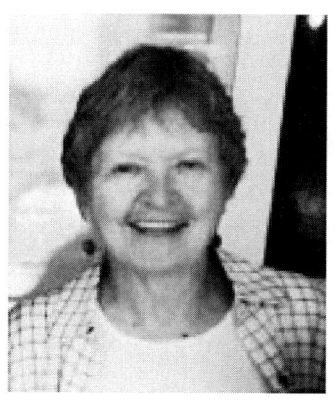

A professional writer and editor with a Master's Degree in Creative Writing, Tessa has published a number of magazine pieces and written well over a thousand articles for *The New York Times*. Living on opposite coasts, we were on the phone a lot. With Tessa I knew I was in good hands. (Her name spelled backwards: Asset!)

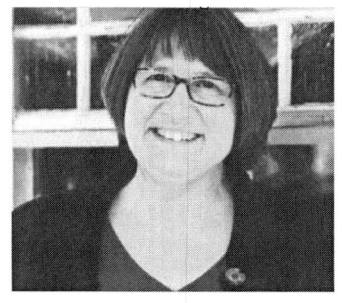

Liz Korabek-Emerson became a fast friend in the last year as we worked on this memoir together. Liz has been in the theatre business for over thirty years and has written and performed a variety of plays. She now teaches mindfulness classes at local colleges and medical facilities. She was instrumental in keeping me organized. She has great patience with my lack of computer skills and continually saved me from my-self. We have a great deal of fun laughing together.

Nancy Grossman, editor and book designer, was a wonderful find. I can't remember who referred her to me, but I'm glad she did. This book was published under difficult and unexpected circumstances.

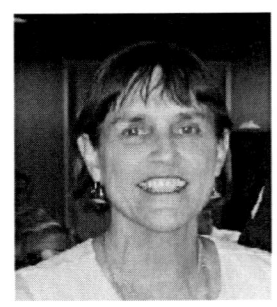

COVID-19 showed up right after my first meeting with Nancy. We weren't able to meet again until more than two months later when Nancy's lock-down where she lived was lifted. She and I, instead, talked by phone and emailed each other about the book. Dealing with COVID-19 was a real disappointment. I wish we could have met more in person.

Nancy was a delight to work with. She was perfect for me, the right fit. Simply amazing. Nancy was low key, kind and patient, particularly as she experienced my Parkinson's symptoms: dropping papers and pens, not being able to write legibly, my ineptness at the computer, and my general slowness. We were held up by both Parkinson's and COVID-19, but neither stopped us. We forged ahead.

Debby Ronnquist, a local artist, painted the watercolor at the end of the color photo section one afternoon sitting on my deck over-looking Chauncey Creek. A well-known member of the Kittery community, she was instrumental in the founding of Fair Tide, whose mission 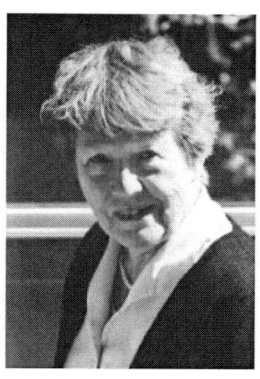 is to reduce homelessness in the Seacoast, then later Fair Tide Thrift Shop and The Fabulous Find, a resale boutique which donates its profits to local non-profit organizations. She was also a founder of Just Us Chickens, an art gallery currently representing over thirty artists, and has been involved in numerous other local organizations and causes.

Contents

Section 6: It Hasn't Gone Away

Section 7: Experiences Along the Way

Appendix

Section 1

My Life Has Changed

More Words Than I Care to Know

"Play the ball where it lies."
— Bobby Jones, a famous golfer on being
diagnosed with a debilitating illness

What is "micrographia?" A mouthful. How about "dyskinesia," "dystonia," "bradykinesia," "cogwheeling," "festination?" A number of mouthfuls.

Twenty-eight years ago, these words were not a part of my being. But then, neither was Parkinson's disease. Today, those words and the scourge they represent describe my body. But they do not define me.

There are other words—"Eldypryl," "Sinemet." "Azilect," "Neurontin," "Amantadine"—all medicines to help my body move. Twenty-eight years ago, I had no reason to have any of these words as part of my vocabulary. But then I was hit with and engulfed by a personal tsunami and the 'surround sound' of medical terms that accom-

3

pany it. In short, Parkinson's has forced me to learn the lingo.

DISEASE? I hate that word. To me, 'disease' means being drastically sick, possibly hospitalized, a condition usually referred to by something unpronounceable. But I was forty-eight years old, and I had just started living.

In my mind, I didn't have a disease. I wasn't contagious. PD wasn't going to kill me. I had a condition, a progressive, degenerative neurological disorder. Yes, I was depressed, and looking back on it, probably severely depressed. But I didn't feel physically miserable the way sick people do. I felt fine—except I was moving kind of slowly. I thought of my condition as slowly rotting away.

All kinds of books describe the science of Parkinson's, so I won't even try. Simply put, we PD victims have a lack of dopamine in our brains. Dopamine—so the med books tell me—is a neurotransmitter that allows our brains to communicate with the muscles in our bodies. (Aha! So THAT'S why I was moving so slowly.) This all takes place in the "substantia nigra," an area of our brains buried deep in the center. That's about as scientific as I get.

Over the past twenty-eight years, I've developed my own way to describe PD. So, here goes: We are all born with a bucket of dopamine in our brains, but we Parkinsonians have a hole in our bucket, and our dopamine is slowly dripping out. I know that's not the way it happens, but that's my image. The children's song with the line, "There's a hole in my bucket, dear Liza, dear Liza," runs through my head.

When about eighty percent of our dopamine has dripped out, symptoms start showing up. This usually hits people diagnosed with Parkinson's disease sometime in their sixties, give or take. In my case, that was a lot of "take." As I said, I was only forty-eight years old.

Looking back on it, I had first noticed my handwriting was developing a mind of its own, and there was nothing I could do about it. I couldn't write clearly, and what I did write was tiny. That's micrographia—one of those words. My brain simply didn't have enough dopamine to do its job.

Though my symptoms didn't show up all at once, my slow walk soon became a shuffle. Trying to stride briskly out of the grocery store one afternoon, I thought I noticed people staring at me. I held my head up and even smiled at people as I shuffled past, thinking, "I'm too young for this." My smile vanished.

If you ask a group of people, "What is Parkinson's disease?" they often respond with a question of their own:

"Is that the disease where you have a tremor?"

So, here's the good news. Despite my quarter century fighting for my life, I've rarely had a resting tremor. It turns out not all Parkinson's looks the same. My right hand does jerk a lot, and especially when I'm trying to do something really important—like measuring sugar for my cookie recipes. Last Christmas, I ended up with a crunchy granular mess on the floor. But the mess got cleaned up, and I got to create more of my still fabulous cookies, making my grandkids (and me) very happy. The person who wasn't happy was my brother, Steve, who at the time was living with me. He had cleaned up more than his share of messes I made. But he likes my cookies.

As my condition has advanced, non-motor symptoms have appeared. These days, I can't decide if I prefer incontinence or constipation. Choking makes eating difficult, spilling is a given, and I do a lot of laundry. Sometimes I change my shirts three times a day. I should buy stock in OxyClean. I just bought a bib, and I often use a spoon.

My voice has become soft and low, and it's tough to talk loud enough so that I can actually be heard. It's especially hard when I'm in a group such as my writing group. I puff through boxing, but in my weekly writing group, I have trouble giving feedback about someone else's work. I want to be able to contribute more than my voice allows. And, in a sense, that's what I'm trying to do here with this book. Give myself more of a voice. I hope you can hear me loud and clear.

My Name is Mopsy

"I've learned that even when I have pain,
I don't have to be one."
— Unknown

My name is Martha. When I was young, I was called "Mopsy," and still am by family and life-long friends. No one in my family knows for sure where the nickname came from. My mother claimed it came from camp, but my camp friends insist that I arrived with the nickname. Regardless of its origin, it's stuck. Just like Parkinson's disease. No doctor has been able to tell me why I have Parkinson's. But it's stuck with me just like my nickname.

I was tapped for the PD club in 1992, while living in New Hampshire. That's more than twenty-eight years ago, more than a quarter of a century—a long time to deal with such a despicable, insidious disease. Early on, I decided to give a name to whatever had taken over my body. I tried

"Mergatroid," an ugly name for an ugly disease. But soon I decided no name was ugly enough. Now I simply call it, "IT."

When I was diagnosed, I was a single parent raising two high-school-aged children, working more than full time in a new career, and exploring life in a new community and state. In the seven years since my marriage had fallen apart, I had gone from being a community college counselor and faculty member to becoming an insurance agent for Mass Mutual. And in that process, I had moved from Vancouver, Washington, to upstate New York, to New Hampshire. Now I live on Maine's magnificent coast. I'm not moving again.

When I learned I had Parkinson's disease, I went into a tailspin. I felt I was running on empty. I had never been despondent before. But, in my defense, I had never had Parkinson's before either.

Parkinson's disease is no fun. Whether you're a person afflicted with it, a caregiver, a family member, or simply an interested individual, I want to share with you how I have lived my life these past twenty-eight years dealing with IT. Although IT's certainly not a pretty disease, Parkinson's is "doable," as they say. And, yes, good can come out of IT. But, did I believe good could come out of

Parkinson's when I was first diagnosed? Don't bet on that.

I felt violated when people hugged me, and whispered, "Oh, Mopsy, you'll adjust. You'll mourn your old self and then just get on with it."

"Hah," I muttered to myself. "These people have no clue what it's like to have such a terrifying diagnosis."

Today, all I want is to share my story, a memoir that will educate readers—not about the scientific aspects of the disease, but about the nitty-gritty daily grind of living with Parkinson's. And, yes, the positives, too, of living with this affliction, and there are some, definitely.

As the years have passed, I have grown more comfortable with my ever-changing body and no longer feel any embarrassment about what I look like to others. I have adjusted and continue to adjust—a possibility which, early on, I couldn't have imagined.

What I hope to do in these pages is to share some of the experiences that have greatly enhanced my life, despite my decrepit being, from climbing Mount Washington three years after my diagnosis, to my safari trip to Africa, one year after that, to buying a house on a tidal creek in Maine. I couldn't possibly do any of those things today.

These vignettes were written, each by themselves, in no particular order. I've tried, however, to group them into some kind of thematic sequence.

So here, dear reader, is my story.

Can It Be?

I'm forty-eight years old, in good shape, and playing lots of tennis, even winning a few local tournaments. Tennis has always been my passion. But once again, I've overdone it. Another pinched nerve. Damn.

The neurologist is short, with dark curly hair and a pleasant smile. She's very businesslike and almost immediately starts running me through the typical tests.

I've had these 'tennis elbow' problems lots of times, but especially in recent years. It doesn't help being just two years this side of fifty. This time around, I figure I have another pinched nerve in my right hand. It's weaker than usual, and my handwriting has become unreadable. So here I am, touching my nose with alternating fingers, and now she's using that little hammer on me. All familiar stuff.

But then she says, "I need you to walk down the hall and back," so I do, feeling a little unsettled. "Good. Now I want to stand behind you so I can pull you backwards." I hesitate. "Don't worry," she says, patting my shoulder. "I'll be sure you don't fall. Now, please stand on one foot with your eyes closed. Good. The other foot?"

Now what? She's got a little flashlight out, explaining she wants to examine my eyes for blinking patterns. But—I've come to see her for a pinched nerve, thank you very much. Reaching over, she lifts my hands and arms and starts moving them around, and then around again.

"You're moving them a lot," I say, ignoring the knot in my stomach.

"Trying to see if there's any cogwheeling effect," she says, her voice brisk. "It's part of the exam, and I like being thorough." She doesn't explain "cogwheeling," and I don't ask.

"One more thing," she says, coming over to the table beside me. "Please write a few sentences and then draw some concentric circles on this paper."

As I'm completing this ridiculous test, I can feel her watching me closely. "How'd I do?" I ask, keeping it casual.

She says nothing, returning to her desk where she fumbles with some papers, then pauses and looks me straight in the eye. "Martha, I think you may have early onset Parkinson's disease."

I go numb. The silence is deafening. The knot in my stomach rises and rises some more. I swallow hard.

"I hope you know I hadn't planned on this being part of my day," I say, my voice weak and far away. I clear my throat and press on.

What IS Parkinson's?

What can I expect?

How is it treated?

What kind of research is going on?

How soon will there be a cure?

Aren't I—too young for this?

I am so matter of fact, I might as well be asking how to grow turnips. When I finally stop to catch my breath, the doctor looks at me for a moment and says in a quiet voice, "Martha, I expect a cure within ten years."

I hold on to her words, finding the strength to reply, "You've put me through the wringer today. And, I'm going to need a second opinion. Can you help me with that?"

"Of course I can," she says, immediately going to her Rolodex and pulling out the names of two physicians specializing in Parkinson's, the people I quickly learn to call "Movement Disorder Specialists." I take her note and rise from my chair, desperate to leave but determined to move smoothly and quickly.

It's only when I get behind the steering wheel that the tears come. This cannot be happening. This must be a bad joke. Parkinson's disease? That's a disease for old men. Isn't it?? That's what Mr. Nevell had, wasn't it? We all loved him, the father of my college friend, Nancy. He always came to our father-daughter weekend even though he shuffled when he walked, his hands shook, and you could hardly hear him or understand anything he said.

I grip the wheel, laying my head against it, hugging it. I loved Mr. Nevell, but I didn't want to be like him, not now, not ever. But sitting here, staring into the emptiness before me, I know I have just pulled the short straw, and my life as I know it is over.

To Boston

"The pessimist sees difficulty in every opportunity.
The optimist sees opportunity in every difficulty."
— *Winston Churchill*

"**Y**ou up for this?" I asked, giving her a quick glance as she drove us south on 95 toward Mass General Hospital in Boston.

"That's what family's for," she muttered softly, staring straight ahead. Susan is my sister, and she had called to say she wanted to take me to Boston for a second opinion—the opinion that would let me know whether I really had contracted this dreadful disease.

Susan had offered to drive the two hundred and twenty-nine miles from Connecticut to my home in Durham, New Hampshire, and take me to this place in Boston, this famous hospital center with a reputation for knowing it all. Sue would drive me back home that night, and after spending the night, drive home to Connecticut the next morning. And she planned to do it two more times. I couldn't believe Susan was willing to give up her time to do this for me. We were only eighteen months apart in age, but we weren't that close. But now I was grateful for her presence, grateful she sensed my fear and my terror.

The Boston skyline suddenly appeared before us. "We're getting closer," I moaned, unable to prevent the words from escaping.

"Try not to jump to conclusions," Sue said, giving me a quick glance. "You really aren't going to know what's going on until we get there."

Walking from the parking garage, Mass General appeared above us, a massive place, overwhelming me with its size. It sits at the end of a narrow street lined with tall buildings. It loomed over us. I felt like I was in a cave, about to walk through those revolving doors to get eaten by some unknown and terrifying creature.

But everybody was walking with purpose so we did too, passing through the entrance doors with ease. Taking the elevator to the eighth floor, we kept up our rhythm, walking to *"our door."*

"So, we're here," I tried to say calmly. But I found myself staring at the brass plaque in front of me. "Multiple

Sclerosis, Stroke, ALS, Parkinson's, Alzheimer's."

It hit me. This is serious business. I don't belong here.

I paused. I started to take a step but hesitated again. Sue looked at me and said quietly, "We need to go in." Holding the door open for me. I took in a big gulp of air and walked into the waiting room.

I was stunned. Susan gave me a glance that told me she knew exactly what I was thinking.

Entering that waiting room put me into a whole new disturbing world. Writhing, shaking bodies, hands with tremors, people drooling, people staring with no expression. Some in wheelchairs. Many with walkers. Without intending to, I found myself staring at these poor people waiting to see their doctors.

Am I going to look like that someday? I don't want any part of it. Now I was damned scared.

I picked up a magazine and thumbed through the pages, but wasn't reading a thing. I felt hollow inside. I picked up a second magazine, then a third, then a fourth. I kept leafing through the pages, not seeing anything. I breathed deeply, trying to relax. Sue sat next to me and held my hand for a brief moment. She reassured me that I would be all right.

There is no definitive test for diagnosing Parkinson's

such as a blood test. The diagnosis comes from clinical observation and ruling out other abnormalities such as a brain tumor. Despite my initial diagnosis, I had convinced myself that a second, and perhaps a third opinion would set things right again, would restore me to sanity and security. Now, looking at these decrepit people, I could hardly breathe.

My first appointment that day included a neurological exam and an Alzheimer's test just to be sure that my brain wasn't screwy and that my memory was okay.

I first met with Marcia Tennis, a nurse practitioner who reassured me that Parkinson's was a "doable" disease—the first time I heard that word—although she agreed, not much fun. She was very calming. A lovely person. Marcia Tennis.

After asking me a bunch of questions, Marcia said I would be perfect for a study involving people diagnosed within the past year. But I haven't even been officially diagnosed at that point, I wanted to say.

Marcia invited Dr. Stephen Fink to meet with us. He was the most relaxed doctor I'd ever met. He listened to everything I had to say. The fact that he was easy to look at didn't hurt at all.

After explaining the study to me, my hope returned.

Dr. Fink asked me a lot of questions, but when he discovered how young I was, he seemed surprised and hesitated. "The company sponsoring the study," he said, "requires that a woman could not have the possibility of getting pregnant."

"Can't you tell them I'm a nun?" I said, hoping a joke would cover my dismay.

My second appointment at Mass General required an MRI to rule out brain tumors and other brain abnormalities. Great. I already had a partially frozen shoulder from a prior injury so it was tough being still for so long while the machine clanked around me. The lab technician got upset with me for moving too much. Lady, you crawl in here and see how still you can be, I felt like saying. She was clearly having a bad day or was perpetually unpleasant. I'd doubt if she knew or cared how I was feeling.

After my MRI ordeal, I met with Dr. John Growden, Department Chair of Neurology at Mass General. He went through the drill. Another neurological exam? Every time I met with a different neurologist, I found myself doing the same things over and over. How many times must I quickly go back and forth, first touching my nose and then the doctor's finger? The answer, I have learned, is: every time, all the time.

The doctor prescribed something called "Sinemet" for me to take for three weeks until my third appointment. "If it works on a trial basis," he explained, "it pretty much means you have Parkinson's disease. Sinemet or Carbidopa/Levadopa," he told me, "is the gold standard for treating Parkinson's." Dr. Growden asked me to notice, during this three-week trial, if my right arm started swinging more naturally, and if I could write more easily and more clearly.

I looked at my sister as we left his office and said quietly, "I'm not sure if I want this medicine to work or not." Susan nodded, squeezing my hand.

During that three-week period, I knew.

When we returned to Mass General for my third appointment, the neurologist said he had both good and bad news for me. The bad news: I had Parkinson's Disease. BAM! Just like that.

The good news? I couldn't possibly imagine there was any good news, but the saving grace was that I didn't have one of the rare Parkinson's-like diseases that doesn't respond to medication. So, this made me lucky? The neurologist explained that there were medications to relieve the early symptoms of Parkinson's. I called it a cover-up because the disease would continue to progress in spite of the medications.

On the way home, I felt empty. I wasn't surprised at the diagnosis. My sister and I traveled in silence. But as we grew closer to home, I couldn't stop the tears from filling my eyes. I continued to cry softly, mourning my former life that was no longer, while Susan held my hand once more.

Section 2

Friends and Family
Learning About Parkinson's

Telling the Kids

"Turn your wounds into wisdom."
— *Oprah Winfrey*

Arriving home after my shattering appointment, I fly upstairs to my room, not bothering to say hello to Stephen and Katie, my teenagers. I always greet them, but today is not always.

I have to be alone. I shut the door quietly, hoping the kids won't notice that something is wrong. I fall onto the bed, burrowing into the pillow now soaking up my tears. Gasping, I lift my head and stare at the walls, but I see nothing. I can't think. I can't breathe. I can't speak. My fear is unimaginable.

Time passes. I find myself on the phone, clutching it to my ear, desperate for my parents, silently wishing them to be with me. Stoic New Englanders, neither of them knows what to say.

"But Mopsy, you are in such good shape. You are such a good athlete." My dad is trying to speak calmly though his voice is unsettled, his shock obvious.

Now Mom comes on. "It won't be so bad," she says, her voice creamy, like butter. "You'll lick it if anyone can. You can handle it."

"*I HAVE PARKINSON'S DISEASE*," I want to shout. But I just grip the phone tighter. Neither of them can deal with my pain. And, I quickly realize, neither can I. What am I to do?

I call a good friend. Another mistake. She holds forth with the same platitudes I got from my parents. After I deal with the shock of it all, I'll just "get on with life," she says knowingly, her voice soothing. Really? She knows nothing. My life as I know it has just been destroyed.

I call another friend. This one just listens. It feels as if she is embracing me right over the telephone wires, hugging me with silent compassion and empathy. She's just what I need.

As my Parkinson's progresses, I will soon learn that there are three kinds of people: those who can talk about "IT," those who won't and those who can't. Same is true for the "big C," or all the rest of these dreaded diseases that strike without warning. The first group shows they care by asking good questions, but best of all, they listen. The second group also cares, but it's clear they can't deal with my reality. And the third group simply walks away.

Two weeks go by while I walk around the house totally numb, my nerve endings raw. My poor children. I can't tell them, not yet, not until I can—in some measure—grasp what is happening to me. During those days, while I am mulling everything over, Stephen, seventeen, and Katie, fifteen, can do nothing right. I am constantly yelling at them. I can attend to them, but I have no mothering in me.

"I have a problem," I finally announce at dinner with a big sigh. "I'd like to talk to both of you right after we finish eating. I'll do the dishes later." My pronouncements, especially my offer to do the dishes, throw a wet blanket over the rest of the meal. This is serious.

We finish eating in silence and file into the living room. I can feel my heart pounding, the sweat forming on my brow. I feel so alone facing them.

"This isn't easy to share," I say, diving in, trying for a brisk tone though my voice is hoarse. "Two weeks ago, I went to a doctor because I thought I had another pinched nerve." Katie and Stephen continue to sit quietly, staring past me, their faces blank.

"But what the doctor told me was quite unexpected and not what I wanted to hear. Seems I have early onset Parkinson's disease." Now I rush on, trying to ignore their faces. "Having Parkinson's isn't such a drastic diagnosis, and I'm not going to die from it." I move on quickly, determined to sound upbeat while holding back my tears. "The majority of cases of Parkinson's are not genetic." I was trying to reassure them—and myself.

"I know about Parkinson's," Stephen says, his voice low but steady, his eyes locked on mine. "I saw it on *Nova*. This is not good, Mom."

I shift in my chair, seeking words that will comfort. "No, it's not good," I say, "but it's a disease that develops gradually. The symptoms won't appear all at once."

Katie has said nothing. In the silence that follows, she gets up and leaves us without a word, walking slowly upstairs. My daughter has trouble dealing with difficult things, just like the rest of my family, but this is a tough one.

I don't realize how tough until a few days later when I wander into her room to drop off some laundry. Her bed has been made with military precision, the first time that's ever happened. Then I notice her diary lying open on her bed. Katie always puts it away, never leaving it out, let alone open. I know the page is for me. "This is the worst day of my life," she writes.

How painful to read these words. I want her in my arms right this minute. But as I stand there while more tears flow, I realize my children have made me aware that Parkinson's isn't just my disease. It's our disease. That hurts. A lot. But I also realize that I am no longer alone.

Telling My Parents

"The family is one of nature's masterpieces."
— *George Satayana*

One of the most painful parts in the beginning stages of dealing with Parkinson's was not being able to talk to my parents easily. Though they were the first ones I called when diagnosed, after that not much was said, except in passing.

I had been dealing with this scary condition for almost nine months when my parents came for their annual summer visit. I decided I wouldn't bring up Parkinson's but would wait for them to bring it up. I realized that I, too, was challenged, afraid to tell my parents just how monumental this felt in my life.

Parkinson's was rarely mentioned.

This couldn't go on. I needed them to realize that Parkinson's was consuming my life. It was out of character for them to reply with silence. With the help of a therapist,

I set a goal for when I was next in Florida: Talk to Mom and Dad about their not recognizing that my life had suddenly been turned upside down.

Six months later I visited my folks in Mt. Dora, Florida. Early in my visit, my mother and I headed out for a walk around one of the lakes near where they lived. It was a warm, pleasant day and both of us wore shorts and T-shirts. Sitting on my mother's head, her white cotton hat shaded her eyes from the sun. It was frayed at the edges like an old friend. My mother would never consider replacing it.

I fixed my eyes on a spot across the lake. If my mother hadn't asked me about my Parkinson's by the time we reached that point, I thought to myself, I am going to ask her why she can't talk about "IT."

As we walked, Mom must have read my mind. "I notice your right arm doesn't swing when you walk," she said. "Is that Parkinson's related? Your left arm seems perfectly fine. Why is that?"

Well, blow me over. We talked a bit about my arm not working. "Stiffness is a significant part of Parkinson's and symptoms usually start on one side of the body. The left side will catch up soon enough." I said the last part jokingly but it suddenly hit me that the cause of the unease with my parents was our having different coping styles. My parents chose silence. I opted for humor. The key thing now was that the barrier had been cracked and was beginning to crumble.

"You don't have a tremor. Maybe you don't have Parkinson's," she said hopefully.

"Mom, not everyone with Parkinson's has a tremor."

We continued around the lake. I held my breath and then said, "Mom, I really appreciate your asking me about my condition. It's been difficult dealing with your silence."

She responded in her best New England style. "Your father has trouble talking about it."

I stopped walking, looked at her directly and said, "Mom, I'm not talking about Dad. I'm talking about you. I need you to recognize that having Parkinson's in my life is a very big deal."

"You want me to ask about it every time we talk on the phone?" she asked.

"Every once in a while would be nice," I said with some sarcasm. I was relieved to be having this conversation.

"Martha, I know your diagnosis has been tough on you," Mom said softly. "I didn't want to bother you about it. You've always been so healthy and active that I can't quite believe it. You know how much I love you. I would never knowingly do something to hurt you, you know that."

"Well, I really appreciate you talking with me. I am frightened by my diagnosis. The ramifications of it are enormous."

Ice clinked in our glasses that night while having drinks before dinner. Any ice between us was being chipped and melted away by conversation. My mother talked about my mother-in-law who had died a few years earlier of breast cancer. "I admired Ruth so much," Mom said. "She was so open in talking about her cancer."

"Mom, you might use Ruth as a role model for openness," I said gently.

Then on to my dad. Just like my mother, I needed him to acknowledge my struggle. Whenever I visited my parents, my father always took me to his local golf club to play a round with his cronies. He always bragged, "You should see my daughter hit the ball."

I remember as a kid going to the golf club with my father on summer evenings. He always threw down extra balls for me to hit. Often, we jumped from hole to hole, usually out of order, depending on how many people were on the course. It was cross country golfing at its best.

Four days after I arrived in Mt. Dora, Dad said, "Let's play golf today."

I said, "Fine," and off we went. Dad was a natural athlete and fortunately I inherited his genes. This gave us shared experiences and fostered a closeness between us. He was a scratch golfer in his prime and was a member of the All-American Collegiate Golf Team way back in 1933. I always bragged about how he shot his age when he was 69, an extraordinary feat for any golfer. But what I needed from him now was a recognition of my struggle with Parkinson's.

As we drove away from the course that warm day in February, I thanked my father for taking me to play, making helpful suggestions, and being patient with me. Dad always hit the ball straight down the fairway. I, on the other hand, too often found myself in what my dad called the tall grass.

After a brief pause in our conversation, I commented, "It's ironic, Dad, that you're giving up golf because of a medical condition, your macular degeneration, while I'm playing more golf than tennis because of a medical condition, Parkinson's disease."

I felt a lump in my throat but continued anyway. "Dad,

I have no idea how you feel about my having Parkinson's. You rarely talk about it."

His voice wavered, and he bit his lip. After a long pause, he cried, "Martha, I'm devastated. I think about it every day. I'm afraid I caused it. I just don't know what to do."

Here was my father, a sensitive, caring man who didn't always know how to bring up sensitive issues, yet this was the breakthrough I was after. Since then, each time we talked, he always asked how I was and I always knew what he meant. I reassured him a number of times that he had nothing to do with causing my Parkinson's.

I miss talking to both of my parents. After that visit, everything changed. They wanted to learn more about my condition, and they always asked how I was feeling. They often sent me news articles about new treatments and promising research, and they made yearly contributions to the Michael J. Fox Foundation and to the Parkinson's Unity Walk. They, along with my kids, became my greatest supporters. In a strange way, the very disease that I felt was ending my life, as I knew it, helped create even a stronger bond with my parents than I could ever have imagined.

For my part, I am more comfortable with my body,

even as the disease progresses. I now have no need to dwell on having Parkinson's, except in writing this memoir. Parkinson's is now in the open, can be easily discussed, and even laughed at.

Telling the World

"No one can make you feel inferior without your consent."

— *Eleanor Roosevelt*

Being diagnosed with Parkinson's is not unlike being identified, handpicked, and dive-bombed by a Parkinson's disease drone. ZAP! My life was changed forever.

I had been blasted into the middle of a swamp. I was standing in quicksand, with friends and family looking on from the periphery. I couldn't move. I avoided people because I wasn't ready to talk about "IT." I was scared and alone. I knew I would be better off if I were open with people, but I couldn't be.

Not yet.

Eventually I lifted one foot, then the other. I began by moving slowly, "slowly" being the operative word. I began by telling people close to me about my diagnosis, but it ended there. I knew my symptoms didn't show early on so I didn't need to talk about it, and yet I believed, mistakenly, that everybody could tell I had Parkinson's. I kept my right hand in my pocket so people wouldn't notice that my right arm was stiff and hung by my side when I walked. Now, when people look at me funny, I think to myself, "So what?"

One day when talking to my friend, Tessa, she said, "You have to meet Jim. I worked with him at *The New York Times*. He's had Parkinson's for a while now, and I know he'd be happy to meet you."

A few months later, I called Tessa. "Set up that luncheon with Jim. I'll be heading towards the Tappan Zee Bridge in two weeks. Stephen and I are going to visit colleges."

We met at a Greek diner in Tarrytown, NY. Jim came in late, went to a bank of phones, and called in a big story he had been working on. From behind, he looked perfectly normal.

Then Jim came to the table. I noticed his rumpled look, wild hair, and coffee stains on his shirt. He had real difficulty eating the Rueben sandwich he ordered and sloshed coffee from his cup to his saucer to the table. Eating was not an easy task for Jim because of his tremor, but I admired that he ordered what he wanted to eat rather than what was easiest to eat. He was very comfortable with his body and didn't apologize for any messes he made. But I felt uneasy.

Was that how I was going to be in a few years?

"Before I was diagnosed," he said, "I came out of my office every morning to greet the journalists and reporters working for me. My door was always open. Once I was diagnosed, I turned into a hermit. I kept my office door closed and brought my morning greetings to an abrupt end. My staff became anxious, wondering what was going on." Later, when Jim finally stopped being a recluse and started talking about having Parkinson's, everyone said to him, "Thank goodness. We were so worried about you hiding away."

When I asked Jim what he would do differently, if he could do it over, he declared, "I would talk to my family, friends, colleagues and acquaintances much sooner. They have been a wonderful support to me, support I could have had earlier if I had been smarter." He looked at me straight in the eye and said, "You have been handed a cruel disease. It's nasty, but it's doable." That word again. "I encourage you to face it head on and don't worry for one minute what people think. But do talk to people. It makes it much easier."

———— // ————

A few months after meeting Jim, with my senses still raw from my diagnosis, I participated in a motivational seminar through work, a follow-up to a seminar earlier that year. I sat with tears in my eyes and my head down except when I stole a look from the man across the table from me. I knew he was watching me. We locked eyes. Both of us quickly looked away. The topic was about improving our lives and setting personal goals. The only thing that could improve my life was getting rid of this despicable disease.

After lunch, Ed, who was my general agent at Mass Mutual, and one of the most sensitive and empathetic men I know, came up to me, gently pulled me away from the other agents and said, "Let's talk. I'm concerned about you. I noticed you were teary eyed throughout the morning."

Ed was not tall, had graying hair and looked good in tweedy sports coats. He exuded a genuine warmth that was very real, very much like a great big teddy bear. When I told him I had Parkinson's, tears flooded his eyes. He cried with me, then said, "Go home for the afternoon. You don't need to walk back into that seminar room again today." I left, but not without a hug from Ed.

One day, Ed said to me, "Be yourself. You are a trusting person. So, trust." I started telling more people about my shocking news but took it slowly. I first began with people I knew who would be compassionate and caring. Then I widened the circle. I got a variety of reactions with most describing an element of surprise.

"You don't look like anything's wrong with you."

"You can't have it. You're far too healthy."

"But you don't have a tremor."

Some changed the conversation to a different topic. A few walked away. The most satisfying interactions were with people who asked questions and were genuinely interested in learning about Parkinson's. I felt like a real person with those folks.

Now, I talk with anyone and everyone about Parkinson's. Unsuspecting people in line at the grocery store, or the bank, people I have just met. My symptoms are quite visible now so I'm very up-front about having Parkinson's. I find that my being open diminishes people's anxiety and keeps folks from wondering. I might as well tell them what it is. I might as well tell the world.

Section 3

Living Fully With PD

Marcye

"The most beautiful people I've known are those who have known trials, have known struggles, have known loss, and have found their way out of the depths."
— Elizabeth Kübler-Ross

I t would never have happened if I hadn't pulled that short straw and ended up with Parkinson's Disease. It would never have happened if Marcye hadn't had breast cancer. Without cancer and Parkinson's looming over us, it's unlikely we would have ever met. But with both of us faced with life changing illnesses, our different journeys shared the same road.

It all began when I called Marcye, an insurance client of mine that I had inherited, to ask some mundane questions about her life insurance policy. As we were taking care of business, the young woman's voice grew faint.

"Sorry, Marcye, I'm having trouble hearing you," I said politely. "Could you speak up a bit?"

"I have breast cancer," she suddenly blurted out, her voice trembling.

"And I have Parkinson's," I replied just as suddenly. I had never, ever mentioned my condition to a client, and now I gripped the phone, staring at it in shocked silence. At that point, I'd had a Parkinson's diagnosis for the past five years.

"I have just the place for you," Marcye's soft voice began again, but this time, sounding steady, determined. "Come to a reiki clinic this coming Wednesday evening. I'll meet you there." And so I met Marcye. I attended the reiki clinic at Portsmouth Hospital for two years. Never would I have guessed I would benefit so much from one phone call.

After our reiki session that first evening, Marcye and I talked some more. What was missing from my life was a sense of community, I told her, and once again she replied, "I have just the place for you." This time it was, "Come to church with me on Sunday." I did not consider her comment proselytizing. I hadn't been to church in years, but somehow her suggestion felt right. I met Marcye at her house that very next Sunday, and off we trotted to the First Congregational Church of Kittery at Kittery Point—the oldest church in Maine.

That first Sunday, I met many wonderful people, starting with Jill, the minister, a very welcoming woman with a delightful sense of humor. I was so taken with the people I met that Sunday that I started going to church there every two or three weeks—even though it was twenty miles away. Soon after that, I decided I wanted to live in Kittery. The kids were off at college, and I had no reason to stay in Durham, New Hampshire, in the town where we had lived when they were in middle and high school.

From then on, it was history. Besides Marcye, numerous other friends in her church encouraged me to move to Kittery. I had never been in such a welcoming place. Marcia Gibbons, a friend from church, called me anytime she heard of a house for sale or possibly for sale. And what did I end up finding? My dream house, of course, a house right on the water, a place where I can see the birds from my deck.

I know my meeting with Marcye and my being introduced to this wonderful church and the people in it was no accident. Something larger than me was involved. My journey had led me to a new and gratifying faith, one that grows stronger each day.

In a strange sort of way, Parkinson's has ended up being a gift. I don't believe God gave me Parkinson's, nor do I enjoy having it. But I do believe God gave me some special gifts to deal with it. Without Parkinson's, I never would have had those two conversations with Marcye which brought me to this church and community. I never would have had the gift of Marcia and all the help she has given me, nor would I have found my wonderfully healing home. I would not have had Jill and the gifts of her ministry. And I never would have had the gift of all the special friends who make up this warm and caring church community. I treasure each and every one of them. God does indeed give us gifts, in many different ways and in many different packages.

Higher Finances

"Happiness is not a matter of events, it depends upon the tides of the mind."

— *Alice Meynell*

The call came one Friday morning while I was at work. Jim, my realtor, had a house for me to see. The owner had died and her son was taking closed bids, the deadline two days away. As Jim described the house, a 100-year-old New Englander in Maine directly on a tidal creek, I felt a joy I thought my Parkinson's diagnosis had killed forever. I had been dealing with "IT" for six years. I had dreamed of owning a home on the New England coast for most of my adult life. But as soon as I heard the asking price, my dream died. "Forget it, Jim," I said, ending our call abruptly. Just as quickly, Jim called back. "You've got to see it, Martha," he said in his low-key but forceful way. I caved in.

A few hours later, we were pulling into the drive. You couldn't see much from the road because of all the lilac bushes about ready to pop. But rounding a curve in the driveway, there it was—this old New Englander with its old wooden deck overlooking a welcoming expanse of clear, sparkling water. The sight left me speechless. But the words came quickly.

"Jim, this is it," I said, one foot still in the car.

Standing on the red-painted porch with its green ceiling, I gaped at the beauty of this spot. The craggy shoreline with its sliver of ocean in the distance was similar to the watercolor my brother, Steve, had given me for my birthday a year ago. The painting, with its gray cape and colorful garden overlooking the water, showed a house surrounded by a white picket fence. This house had no picket fence, but I didn't need one.

The creek had a certain intimacy, Jim observed, watching me gaze at this magical scene, its tides tied to Pepperell Cove. The difference between low and high tide? Ten to twelve feet, he continued, though he knew I wasn't listening. I would soon learn that this tidal waterway was a favorite of kayakers and rowers with the rower's boathouse directly across from my deck, a place I had no idea would become famous for my gin and tonic parties.

The house itself was less important to me than the location, but when I finally went inside, I liked what I saw. Every room except the downstairs bath had a view of the water, and if you left the door open to the bathroom, you had a view there too. Did the house have a furnace? A septic tank? I had no clue, but it didn't matter.

So what do you do when you want a house you can't afford? I had to do some creative financing. My dad was good with financial matters, so the minute I got home, I called him, barely able to contain my excitement. To my surprise, he came up with all kinds of reasons why I shouldn't buy the house.

"You can't afford it." True. "You'll have to sell your house in New Hampshire, and it's not a good time to sell." Also true. "You have Parkinson's. Buying this house in Kittery would put too much pressure on you financially, physically and emotionally. It takes a lot to move."

My dad missed the most important truth of all: From the moment I had first laid eyes on this house, I knew it was a healing one, that it would be calming and good for my soul. I knew my dad was being protective of me, and I appreciated his concern. I also knew I wasn't going to take his advice.

Fortunately, I had taken some preliminary steps before I had started to look for a house. The most important one? Hooking up with Jim, the realtor, who came highly recommended. Since Jim knew about my financial situation, as we left Kittery and drove out of the driveway, I asked if he truly felt I could handle buying this dream come true.

"I wouldn't have called you if I didn't think that," Jim said, giving me a wink. "And Martha, you've done something most people don't think about—you've gotten a pre-approved loan. The terms of a sales agreement can be just as important as the sale price." Yup, I had seen my mortgage officer even before I met with Jim.

I have always been a saver. My father taught me well. Because of his advice through the years, I managed to figure out a way to buy my house on Chauncey Creek, even though he had been against the idea. So how did I do it?

I discarded the idea of selling the kids to the highest bidder, but I did put together a potpourri of more practical strategies. Along with my initial offer on the house, I included a personal letter. "The house reminds me of our grandmother's old family place in Moody, Maine. Even more importantly, now that I am dealing with the effects of Parkinson's and not leaving the house as much, it's become essential that I have a home and surroundings that would offer me such joy and peace."

I cashed in part of my life insurance policy. I cashed in savings, including some retirement accounts. I could do this knowing I had a long term care policy, giving me some comfort and security for the future. One month later, the house was mine. It was 1998. The house had been built in 1898.

Back in New Hampshire, the housing market dropped— just as Dad said it would. So right after I bought my house on Chauncey Creek, I rented out my home in Durham. In the three years to come, that market would rebound, making it possible to get a higher price for that house— which I did.

As I was working through all my financial shenanigans, I told my parents nothing. Since they had warned me against buying the house, I knew they would just stew about it until they came for their summer visit two months hence. My brother, Steve, picked them up at the Boston Logan Airport, having made up some tale as to why he was driving to Kittery.

Driving down the driveway, the sparkling water in view, my father exclaimed, "Who lives here?" As I walked out onto the porch, a gigantic smile on my face, my parents were stunned. "This is spectacular," my mother gasped. We celebrated well that evening with cocktails and dinner on the deck.

Every day my father sat in his special corner of the deck, looking straight down the creek and said things like...

"This is the best thing you've ever done."

"You amaze me. You pulled this off perfectly."

"I'm so glad you didn't listen to me."

The tide goes in and the tide goes out, the landscape, bird life, weather and light constantly changing. At high tide, I experience the fullness of the creek with a little rock formation down from my newly purchased property mostly covered with water that reemerges as the tide goes out. Nothing is ever the same and yet it is the same. The constant is change.

The beauty of my home is that it is one with nature. Wherever I look, I'm looking outside, looking at a creek that is integral to the house. I look at a body of water with immediacy and an intimacy that soothes my soul and a sight that continues to make having Parkinson's bearable.

The Miniature Bathtub

"If you stumble, make it part of the dance."

— Unknown

When I had a leak in my downstairs bathroom shower that required a lot of work, I needed to use the upstairs bathroom as a backup. The problem was that the upstairs bathroom had a tub, but no shower, due to the angled roof line. The tub was also small and crammed into a tight space. The last time I had used it, about a year earlier, I had had difficulty getting out of it. Common sense told me that it would be even more difficult a year later since improvement of symptoms was not the nature of Parkinson's disease. Nevertheless, I forged ahead. I'd had Parkinson's for only seven years. I could do this.

What was I thinking?

After filling the tub, I stepped into it, not very gracefully. Plopped is a better word. Tsunamis hadn't been in the news at this point, but I nearly created one. I was enjoying the warmth of the water when I reminded myself why I was there—to get clean. Once that mission was completed, I pulled the plug and prepared to get out.

I found rather quickly that I no longer could pull myself up and out of the tub by pulling on the low half wall at one end of the tub like I used to. Instead, I needed to turn over and face the other way. To my horror, I got stuck. My knees were jammed in on one side and my bottom on the other. I couldn't move, wedged in like a large hunk of meat in a crock pot. I wiggled and struggled in the now waterless tub, feeling my skin shrivel, turning into the proverbial prune. I was cold. Frustration was mounting. I was in a precarious position, scared and naked.

How long was I going to be stuck? Was anyone going to find me? And who?

With a great reach across the room, I pulled a bath towel from a towel rack into the tub to gain traction. After extreme effort, I finally unstuck my legs and managed to turn the other way. Not a pretty picture.

But then what to do?

After what seemed like forever, I was finally able to grab a bar on the opposite wall, hoist myself up onto the edge of the tub, and dump myself on to the floor. I was on my back, feeling very much like a large beetle that had flipped over, furiously kicking her legs in her bid to get onto her many feet. I finally rolled over onto my knees and, with more effort, miraculously managed to get upright.

I measure the progression of my Parkinson's disease by the things I can no longer do. It's always scary to find another roadblock that adds to that growing list. I'm constantly testing myself, mostly to my detriment and the detriment of the stress levels of those around me. I'm a slow learner when it comes to changing my ways. This time I should have considered other options. Like bathing at a friend's house. Or, staying dirty.

Squeezing the Lemons

"A day without laughter is a wasted day."
— Unknown

Marcia was going to the supermarket to pick up a few items and invited me along. As we walked across the parking lot, she striding, me shuffling from the Parkinson's disease that had been with me for almost fifteen years now, she turned towards me with her usual bright smile and said, "Why don't you use one of those motorized scooters today? It would be perfect for you."

"Are you crazy?" I blurted, as I waved one shaky arm around the parking lot. "I've never used one before, and the store is as crowded as I've ever seen it. You do know it's Thanksgiving in two days, don't you?"

"You can do it," she countered, smiling in her enthusiastic, encouraging way. Marcia has always been my cheerleader. Before I could stop her, she had fetched a scooter from an employee and was riding it towards me with a big grin. The employee raced along beside her and then helped me step into the cart. After giving me a quick explanation of the controls—most of which I failed to take in—he hustled back inside. It was twenty degrees outside.

I took a deep breath and took off. "Hey, this is fun!" I yelled to no one in particular. For the first time in a long time I felt a sense of freedom, being liberated instead of limited. But that nice grocery store clerk had failed to tell me how to control my speed. Or maybe I wasn't listening.

I burst into the dairy aisle where I almost dropped a carton of eggs, and picked up two containers of yogurt while knocking over eight others. The display of the good cheeses presented an obstacle for me. I was able to rest my scooter against the shelf, but I couldn't reach far enough into the refrigerated bin to get the brie I wanted. A young pregnant woman, tattoos on either arm, reached in and handed me what I was wanting and gave me a wide smile. I thanked her.

Cranberry sauce... coffee... seltzer... pasta... Shoppers in each packed aisle jumped aside as I went rushing up and down, swiping a few people as I careened by, crashing into a couple of displays, actually pushing a display of crackers across the end of an aisle. "Joyride" had taken on a whole new meaning. My newfound freedom had given me an entirely new perspective on my limited life.

In the produce section, a nice man stopped me from sending oranges crashing to the floor. "You're having a good time with that thing, aren't you?" he said, a friendly glint in his eyes.

"Yes, my maiden voyage," I replied happily. "But I have Parkinson's, you see, so I don't have much control, and that *is* a little scary."

"Better be careful," he said as he continued to smile. We both had a good laugh.

Marcia was nowhere to be seen so I decided I'd pick up just a few more items and then head for the checkout. Broccoli, mushrooms and romaine made it into my cart.

The last thing I needed was lemons, for what I don't remember. A short, plump woman, wearing an old wool skirt from the nineteen-fifties, was standing smack in front of the lemon display, squeezing and smelling every lemon in the place. After waiting for what seemed forever, I nudged my cart next to her so I could grab a few. Suddenly, just then she stepped right in front of me and BAM! I collided right into her. It was then that I noticed her white cane. *I had driven into a blind person.*

Worse yet, as she turned around to growl at me, I

recognized her. We had met before—at her home of all places. Her brother, Jim, who also had Parkinson's, was visiting from Arizona, and good old Marcia had driven me to the woman's home to meet her brother and trade Parkinson's stories.

What to do? What to say? I was mortified. *How to apologize? I couldn't even remember her name.*

"I'm sorry," I murmured quietly as I edged away from the lemons, hoping to disappear. I did not want this woman to recognize me. Then I remembered... She couldn't see me. Relieved, after grabbing a few lemons, I motored towards the front of the store. I wanted to leave quickly since I was afraid I would be arrested for a hit and run. Marcia and I met up in two different checkout lines and then headed to her car.

"You won't believe it." I said, still shaken.

"What did you do this time?" Marcia asked, staring at me, her worry clear. "Are you okay?"

I was fine, I said, but as I filled Marcia in on my grocery store adventures, with all their joy and pain, we both began to chuckle. Soon we were laughing hysterically. It wasn't funny... but it was.

In a Stupor

"Do the best that you can in the place
where you are, and be kind."
— *Scott Nearing*

"Take one of these before bedtime," my doctor said. "You'll sleep a lot better." I'd had my Parkinson's diagnosis for over fifteen years.

"Good," I said, not asking any details about the drug, accepting it as the panacea I needed. I took the pill as directed. The next morning, I felt drowsy and generally out of it, a discomforting feeling.

"Throw those pills out. It's not worth the risk of taking them," my ninety-seven-year-old mother urged me on the phone later that day. Instead, I tucked the pills into my dresser—in case I might want to try them again sometime. A few months later, after many sleepless nights, I dug through my underwear drawer to find the container. I swallowed the pill for the second time. Ambien.

When I gained a slight bit of awareness early that next morning, a Saturday, it was still dark. I was on the floor, on my stomach, lying next to my bed. My body had totally twisted around, with my head pointed toward the end of the bed and my feet where my head should be.

How did this happen? How did I fall to the floor without waking up? How could I turn around?

I couldn't get to the phone, which was behind me. There was only eighteen inches between the wall and the side of my bed and I was stuck between the two.

I hurt. My neck was so tight that I couldn't turn it either right or left. My face was smushed into the floor. I kept trying to get to the end of the bed, moving a fraction of an inch at a time. By the time I made it, the sun was coming up.

I grabbed for the bookshelf, then the dresser, and then the foot of the bed, each, in turn, to help me stand. When I couldn't get up, I knew something was terribly wrong. I flipped onto my back.

I was scared. It was Saturday, a day my friends typically spent with their families.

What if they don't find me until Monday?

The floor was hard. I was cold. My bladder was full. I stayed in this position for several hours until I found myself in a sea of warm pee. RELIEF. I even fell asleep for a few minutes.

"Martha, are you there?"

"Igor," I screamed over and over. He kept calling my name as well. He was used to my being at home and the doors unlocked. He had come to finish an outdoor project he had done for me. It amounted to screwing two screws into a railing. He called my name again. I screamed back, "IGOR," as loud as I could. I heard his truck door close. He couldn't hear me and drove off. I was devastated.

A few hours later I heard the voice of another friend. My friend Debby. She had never stopped by my house un- announced, let alone on a Saturday. I called her name. I screamed her name. She couldn't hear me and drove off. Again, my hopes were dashed. I have never felt so totally alone.

Why couldn't these friends hear me?

It was then that I realized that even though I thought I was screaming loudly, it was more than likely that my soft Parkinsonian voice had interfered with what I had hoped would be a rescue. I started working my way into the bathroom. I remembered the handle on the side of the bathtub and reasoned that if I could reach that handle, I could pull myself up. I was still on my back and could hardly move. Somehow, I managed to reach the handle.

It had been fourteen hours but I had made it.

I was up.

I sat on the side of the tub for a while until I heard a voice. "Martha, are you there?" This time the voice came from within my home. Three friends had descended on my house and quickly came upstairs to find me. They found me a mess, somewhat unsteady, and still in a fog. "Let's put some dry clothes on you and then we'll get you something to eat." The scrambled eggs and toast they made for me was as good as the Queen's table.

"Let me explain how A.M., Morgan, and I found you," Debby said. "After stopping by, I wondered why you weren't home. I called A.M. to see if you had gone away for the weekend. When A.M.'s response was 'she should be home,' we all rushed over. Morgan had a key." My friends stayed with me a long time, until they felt I was okay. It was dark when they left.

The lesson to be learned: listen to your mother. And have good friends.

A Dark Night

"What lies behind us and what lies before us are tiny matters compared to what lies within us."
— *Ralph Waldo Emerson*

Two a.m, and I still couldn't close my eyes, still couldn't turn off my brain. Wonder how much longer I will even have a brain. Humph.

Only four more days until I would be heading to Baltimore to be evaluated for "Deep Brain Stimulation," as this new and iffy procedure was called. But the docs still had to decide if I even qualified for having electrodes stuck in my brain to slow down the symptoms of this dreadful disease on the verge of taking over my life.

Life? But what if I died? DBS could kill me, the doctor said, adding "Death is an option." Did I really want to risk my life for the sake of jerking less and walking normally? In the middle of the night, I was terrified.

A sudden crash rattled the house, interrupting my dark thoughts. I lay in bed, holding my breath, listening, trying not to jerk, trying to hold still. I heard scratching and a wrestling noise. But it wasn't an animal. It was coming from Steve's bedroom.

I pulled myself up as best as I could, stumbling down the hall, pounding on my brother's door. No response. Pushing the door open, I saw him lying on the floor, gasping and struggling to get up. I couldn't help, but as I watched, Steve managed to pull himself up onto his bed. Cradling his head in his hand, he muttered, "Oh, my God. Oh, my God."

Sitting down next to him, I put my arm around his shoulders and gently asked, "Steve, what is your name?" Pulling his head up, he stared at me with glassy eyes, saying nothing. Reaching for the phone with shaking hands, I dialed 9-1-1.

The emergency crew came quickly, me still in my pajamas. Once they took over with Steve, I put on some clothes as fast as I could for what I knew would be a long night and day at the hospital.

The paramedic and I had quite a conversation on the way to York Hospital. Steve was lucid enough to refuse them putting an IV in. He kept saying, "No, no, no." The paramedic asked me if he was refusing treatment for religious reasons. I told him that Steve just didn't like western medicine. I smiled inside because Steve still had enough spunk in him to live by his values.

Into the emergency room we went. There I saw Steve refuse an IV from one of the nurses. He kept ripping it out. I finally took him by the shoulders, leaned over him so I was face to face with him, and said in a loud voice, "STOP BEING LIKE OUR FATHER." He smiled and started cooperating.

But he grabbed at another opportunity. The doctors and nurses left the room for a quick moment. Steve suddenly got off the table and looked like he was starting to walk out. Well, that was good, I thought to myself. Steve could stand and move his legs. As I shouted for the doctor, he came tearing in and yelled for the nurses to help him since he was a smaller man. Steve was 6'5" and strong.

Off to the intensive care unit we went, a place I hope never to need. Steve by now couldn't talk, although he could still make noises about treatment. They gave him some sedation to calm him down.

As I held my brother's hand, I watched my left leg beginning to shake uncontrollably. It was only then that I realized I had forgotten to take my medication. But should I care at a time like this?

Once he was settled, and I have no recollection of the time frame, I called my friend Marcia for a ride home. I needed to grab Steve's wallet, his insurance card and my address book, to make phone calls to family members. And take my forgotten medication.

As Marcia drove me home, I suddenly remembered my upcoming trip to Baltimore. It had been hard to get an appointment for my DBS evaluation, and terrified though I was, I knew those doctors at the Johns Hopkins Medical Center were the best. But how could I leave Steve? It was clear he had suffered a stroke.

"You're going," Marcia told me flatly. "Martha, of course you're going to go. You can't take care of Steve. You can only take care of yourself, and you will. Steve has a lot of friends around, and he'll be fine."

I did go to Baltimore, I did have the four-day evaluation for DBS. and I did qualify for the procedure. And, yes, It was a success. That surgery has had an immeasurable impact on my symptoms and on my life—as, dear reader, you can tell as you continue reading this book.

Riding home with Marcia at the end of this dark night, all I could think about was my brother. Would he really be okay? And what would I do without Steve to help me out? When my brother had first asked me if he could move in with me as he began his environmental graduate program nearby at Antioch College, in Keene, New Hampshire, I had hoped he could also help me out as my Parkinson symptoms got worse.

Fortunately, Steve's stroke caused minimal physical damage, mainly aphasia, a language disorder that caused him not to be able to communicate. Our brother Bobby helped out as well, flying across the country from his home in Spokane, Washington, shortly after Steve's stroke, to help look after him.

And yes, Steve does have lots of friends in the area, and Bobby helped establish a schedule for them to help out. For the next year or so, each helper picked a morning or afternoon when they could help my brother relearn to speak, read, spell and do math again. Steve is well liked.

As my Parkinson's did get worse, and Steve got better, he was able to help me, scraping me off the floor a number of times as my falls increased. Steve was the farmer of the house, growing vegetables in the summer and fall and attending to the raspberry patch. He also took over the cooking and he is, after all, better at it than I will ever be. I could not have stayed in my own house without him.

It was serendipity that about the same time as I began to require full time care and needed Steve's bedroom for a caregiver, a house came on the market that met his needs. Now my brother lives just a few miles away and comes to see me often. He always gives me a hug and a kiss—but not during COVID, of course—and we share the joys of being alive together.

This athletic brother of mine had suffered a stroke, yet another example of the "what ifs" in life that we are seldom prepared for—and oh, they do keep coming.

Section 4

A New Life

Deep Brain Stimulation

Johns Hopkins Medical Center
January 17, 2008

Life shrinks or expands in proportion
to one's courage."

— Anais Nin

I was lying on the operating table with my head screwed into the table, part way through deep brain stimulation surgery. I was awake, and I had to stay awake through the whole procedure. Looking at the clock, which I wish I hadn't, I saw it was only 11:00 a.m. I was told this whole thing took about nine hours, and I was only three hours into the procedure. This was elective surgery?

Was I nuts for volunteering? Whose idea was this any-way?

Everyone said I had courage. I didn't see myself as

having a choice. It was either turn my brain over to some neurosurgeon or face an increasingly debilitating life. But it had taken me two years to make that decision. At one appointment, I said to the neurologist, "I don't take brain surgery lightly."

"That's good," she said. "You shouldn't."

It was January 17, 2008. I had been living in an increasingly debilitated body for the past fifteen years.

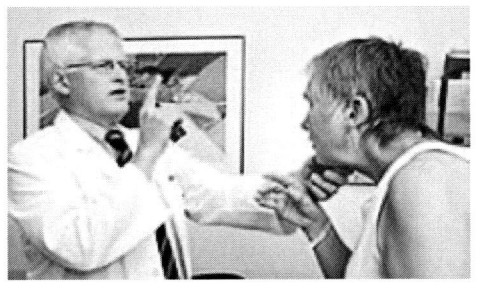

"Good morning," said Dr. Lenz. "We're in for a busy day."

Dr. Frederick Lenz, my neurosurgeon at Johns Hopkins Medical Center, had come into my room at 6:30 a.m. where my kids were waiting with me.

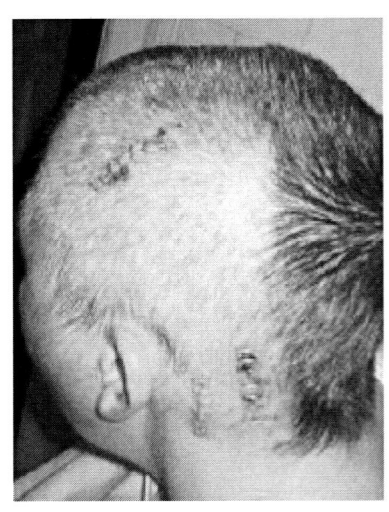

He quickly shaved the front part of my head. I was told later I looked like Clarabell of Howdy Doody fame. This was no beauty shop.

Before this moment, I needed

to be approved for this elective surgery. Two months before, I had to go through all
kinds of testing. I had met
with a speech therapist, occupational therapist, physical therapist, and a psych-
ologist who put me through
four hours of psychological

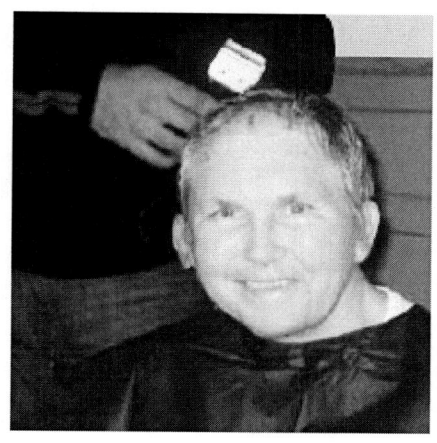

testing and evaluation. I also spent a day meeting with my
neurologist, Dr. Zoltan Mari, a teddy bear of a man from
Hungary, and Dr. Lenz, my neurosurgeon, a slightly built
man who makes up for it with his extensive knowledge.

"Putting on the head gear is the worst part of the
procedure," Dr. Lenz reminded me. "It's the only part that
hurts." He gave me several shots of Novocain in the scalp,
which felt very similar to the time I disrupted a nest of
yellow jackets a few years back.

Dr. Lenz next screwed the headgear into place with
four screws. That hurt. The screws made such indentations
into my scalp that afterwards they looked like mini-craters,
like when I saw Mount St. Helens erupt.

Once my head was encased in the titanium frame, my
two kids continued encouraging me the whole way. I was
surprised how quickly Dr. Lenz whisked me away, the kids

running down the hall trying to keep up with him. "May I take a picture of my mom?" Katie said, sounding exasperated.

"We're having brain surgery today," he retorted. "No photo ops. Quickly say goodbye to your mother."

Quick hugs. "I love you." The elevator doors closed.

Down to the bowels of the hospital. We were in the basement. No special decor here. Nondescript walls, painted pipes on the ceilings, bright lights.

Certain things had to be done before the actual surgery. The titanium frame we could cross off the list. Next, the MRI. Or, I should say MRIs. The technicians shoved me into that machine three times. This, of course, after they screwed my head into the MRI table.

The doctors needed clear images for the next step, mapping the brain. Because of the delicacy of the surgery, mapping the brain was crucial to its success. It was taking longer than usual to complete the process because the computer program they had just put into place was not working properly. Sorry, but they would have to revert to the old program, I was told. I was not feeling comforted. Finally, the operating room was ready for us, and we for them.

Then I heard this horrendous, ear piercing noise, much

like a jackhammer trying to make its way through cement. I realized they were drilling into my head, and I couldn't feel a thing! Dr. Lenz was right. The drill went into my head making a clunking noise. Then it went further. I wasn't prepared for such a noise. A dentist's drill purrs in comparison.

The doctors chit-chatted throughout the procedure, talking about couples going through divorce, books they were reading, the cars they wanted to own, movies they'd seen lately. Clearly, these doctors considered this surgery routine. I didn't. I made myself and my poor clunking brain think of my supportive friends in Kittery and my family. I had to get through this for them.

"Where is that instrument I asked to have at the ready?" I heard Dr. Lenz say in an irritated voice. "I'm angry that things weren't set up properly... I'm just going to do it manually."

Yikes. Please, God, have him know what he is doing.

"We're getting to the important part now," he said, his voice calm but penetrating. "I need you to be as alert as possible. I'm going to touch different parts of your brain with an instrument and I want you to tell me how you feel. Do you feel tingly? Any numbness? Pain? Please move your arms up and down, one at a time. Does this position feel better than the previous one? Now your legs. Do you have any unwanted effects? Let's work with your speech. Any slurring when I touch this spot. Your speech sounds better with the first try."

Dr. Lenz could make my arm tremble or be perfectly still. He could affect my speech, just by moving the instrument to a different spot. It was surreal. "We're going to do the left side of the brain first, then the right side," he said. Then he did.

By the time we got to the right side, I was exhausted. I was ready for it to be over. I was yearning to see my kids.

Stephen and Katie were ecstatic to see me. They had been told that someone would keep them informed of the progression of my surgery, but that hadn't happened. They had been waiting for hours with no news.

ONE WEEK LATER

Now for the part that was going to make everything worthwhile. The second surgery, a week later, was to insert the neurotransmitter device into my chest.

I had to be at Johns Hopkins by noon. I went into the operating room at 2:00 p.m., was in recovery by 4:00 p.m., and back at Stephen's apartment two hours later. I called it Drive-Through Brain Surgery. I had gone under general anesthesia. Much better than staying awake for the procedure.

Dr. Lenz waited three weeks before programming the neurotransmitter because he wanted to take advantage of the residual effects of the surgery. For me that included my walking better and feeling more control of my body. Dr. Lenz's approach to DBS, deep brain stimulation, was very conservative, but that's what I wanted. My dyskinesia (jerky body) all but disappeared and only slightly bothers me now.

Try as I wanted to minimize things, there were very real risks to be considered about this surgery. The big one was death. That was too big to comprehend, though I did sometimes find myself thinking about it in the middle of the night. There were other real risks: getting the electrical leads implanted in the wrong spot, bleeding in the brain, infection, deterioration of speech, balance being affected. But even so, deep down, I had trouble accepting the possibility of something going wrong.

Without surgery, my life would have continued to shrink, shrink, and shrink some more. With surgery, my life had started to expand instantly. I could walk more easily, I could get dressed without a struggle, I had more energy, I could write more legibly, I could drive again, and I could drink red wine again without flinging it all over the place. I no longer needed my two wine sippy cups that are perfectly designed for people with dyskinesia.

It has been twelve years since my initial surgery. Some symptoms have returned. My handwriting is lousy again. I have terrible trouble with balance. I know my body will continue to deteriorate and that my symptoms will increase. But things would have been worse if I hadn't gone through the surgery and I don't regret my decision even though it wasn't a magical cure.

Thanks to Friends

Written after DBS Surgery, Early Spring 2008

A thank you to good friends, Marcia, A.M., Sara and Morgan, for helping me so much and for being such wonderful support to me. They are very special people.

Dyskinesia, dystonia, all these words that I know.
Holes drilled in head, brain surgery to go.
First surgery awake, it was a long day,
But it went really well or so they all say.

Surgery number two was truly a breeze.
I was out for the count, thank you, please.
Completely wired I am, electrodes in brain.
And for this I traveled from the State of Maine.

John Hopkins for me was the way to go
I needed a surgeon who was in the know
Bionic woman, remote in hand,
DBS surgery I say now was quite grand.

Turn me up, turn me down, one click or three
Or stay where it's set and just let it be.
The cards you gave me were simply the best.
The one-a-day brand, I obeyed your request.

They kept me going during my five-week stay.
I could feel your love though far, far away.
You've driven me to doctors, to walking, to church.
Ne'er have I ever been left in the lurch.

You opened my mail, tossed the junk, paid my bills,
And earlier rescued me from Ambien ills.
You've cared for Papi any number of times.
I just can't think of what here best rhymes...

I've got a new lease on life, I don't jerk all the time.
No sippy cup needed for drinking red wine.
Without you, dear friends, it could not have been done.
For the support you gave me I thank you a ton.

Section 5

Was This the Beginning?

I Used to Be Good

"If opening your eyes, or getting out of bed, or holding a spoon, or combing your hair is the daunting Mount Everest you climb today, that is okay."
— *Carmen Ambrosio*

Sometimes I want to wear a sign around my neck reading, "I USED TO BE GOOD." Before Parkinson's hit when I was only forty-eight, I felt strong, confident and accomplished, and I was. I dream about that sign—advertising my considerable athletic abilities—now shrouded in my stooped body, my shuffle, and my pitifully poor balance.

During elementary school I used to play baseball with the boys. A father of one of my classmates, Joe's father, was so impressed with my abilities that he invited me to join his local team. In the 1950s it was unheard of for girls to be involved in boys' sports. Not in Poughkeepsie, New York, my hometown, or anywhere else in the country.

I played better than his son, he told my parents and me. I was so proud and amazed at this father's support. I remember my grandmother one summer in Maine, driving down a dirt road which ended in a playing field. The boys were practicing for their next game. She told me to hop out and go play with them. "You're better than all of them." She was right but I was too shy to leave the car. But, because my family spent summers in Maine, I couldn't commit to playing for the Little League season.

Years later, I was able to see my niece, Julie, play little league in Dover, New Hampshire. Julie was the only girl on the team. I attended as many games as I could. She was my hero!

Back in the old days, girls' basketball had very specific rules, different from the boys. We could only take two dribbles before getting rid of the ball. But the boys? As many dribbles as they wanted. And we girls were either guards or forwards, with each player forced to stay on her half of the court—guards on one half, forwards on the other half.

By the time I had reached eighth grade, I could run the full length of the basketball court faster than most boys I knew, and I could stand it no longer. "Why do the boys' teams get all the attention?" I asked my gym teacher, "and why do the rules for girls insist we must just be ladies? We're athletes, too." I was ready for Title Nine long before it was even a thought to fight for.

But the sport I loved the most was tennis. I had my Dad's natural athletic ability, and I picked up tennis—and golf—easily. Kathe, my best friend growing up, and I played tennis as often as we could—as early in the spring as possible and as late in the fall as we could withstand the cold and the approaching winter. I carried my love of the game straight into adulthood.

Shift to middle age and the lightning bolt that knocked me sideways when I learned I had Parkinson's disease. Before PD, my friend Linda and I had taught tennis together for a number of years at Singing Eagle Lodge. My friends and I spent our summers together at Singing Eagle back in the 1950s and '60s. We bonded well. Our age group and the generation below us now run the camp. Even after my diagnosis I went to visit during the summer.

"I want to see if I can still hit a tennis ball," I said to my friend Linda who agreed to go up to the courts with me just before dinner.

Such was the beginning and end of my tennis career with Parkinson's. I had picked up my racquet again because eight months earlier, I'd had deep brain stimulation surgery. I was no longer flailing all over the place and I could move more easily. I felt like a new person and was certain that my trip back to the courts would be a great success. I hadn't played tennis for a long time, since my game had been reduced to rubble by Parkinson's. I remembered my younger years when I was constantly playing after school during the spring, summer and fall, whenever I could. I played in many local and camp tournaments, winning a number of them. Ah, nostalgia.

Playing with Linda that day, for a few brief moments, I felt almost invincible. It felt so good and so natural, being on a tennis court again. I puffed out my chest like the chickadees in my pear tree at home because I was so proud of myself for hitting the ball and hitting it so well.

My exuberance didn't last long. We'd been playing for about five minutes when Linda hit a blistering shot that came too close to me. I stepped back to whack the ball to her. I stepped back some more. I started taking tiny steps backwards. I couldn't stop. I was going down. Festinations.

I landed full force on my left wrist. I looked down to see it dangling like a dead deer hanging from a tree limb. It would take a plate and eight screws to put my wrist back together again. I felt like Humpty Dumpty.

Linda came running to me, as did our friend Lynn, who had come up to the courts to watch us play. Linda was screaming, "What have I done to you?" To this day, Linda tells me she's sorry for what had happened.

Lynn was the camp nurse that summer. She whisked me off to the hospital right away, confirming gently what I already knew. "It doesn't look good, Mopsy. When you do something to yourself or when something happens to you, you surely do it big. Like Parkinson's. And breaking your wrist."

"I don't want to disappoint."

"No chance of that," Lynn teased me.

With my pathetic-looking wrist propped up on a pillow, I looked up at Lynn and added, "I can't believe it. I'd been doing so well. I was so focused on hitting the ball that it didn't occur to me that I might fall."

"Mopsy," Lynn said, "It makes perfect sense that you did what you did. You were just trying to recreate your old self. That's perfectly normal for someone like you who is such a natural athlete. For God's sake, you must have been on every camp team that Singing Eagle ever had. Didn't you win the tennis cup two years in a row?

"I know it's tough on you being so limited," Lynn said. "It's also tough on your friends. We all hate that you have Parkinson's. You need to know that whether or not you have a broken wrist and whether or not you have Parkinson's, you are dearly loved."

Lynn's words brought the tears on. "I know that," I replied, squeezing her hand with my good one. "I feel so fortunate to have you all in my life." I had finally realized that, sadly, I needed to hang up my racquet. Another loss because of my Parkinson's, but at least I tried. Everyone who knew me well felt the same. "We're proud of you," was echoed over and over, even by the younger campers.

After fighting Parkinson's for the past quarter century —and more—my limitations are severe. But I still hate to see an empty tennis court.

Was This the Beginning?

"Never regret a day in your life. Good days give you happiness and bad days give you experience."

— *Unknown*

"*O*H, MY GOD." *I'm flying through the air. Not good.*

I remember nothing after that fleeting moment. Later a kind person got me to safety and called the police. I didn't know anything. My name, age (twenty-two), where I was living, telephone numbers, nothing. I had no identification on me, no money. I don't even remember talking to the police or the kind person who found me.

I started coming to.

What's this cold plastic I'm sitting on? How did I get here? My mind was one big fuzz ball.

I vaguely remember my friend, Mary, coming up to the window of the police car and asking me, "How are you?" I probably said something inane like, "Just fine."

"What happened to me?" I asked. Mary told me I was in an accident on my bike, and went over the handlebars.

As she talked to the police officer, I heard her say, "When Martha didn't show up within a few minutes, I got worried. She's staying with me temporarily. She's just moved here from the East Coast to La Jolla and started working for the Dean of Students at University of California San Diego one week ago."

Mary was an imposing woman. She was at least six feet tall and, with her deep voice, spoke with authority. She easily convinced the police officer that he could turn me over to her. He seemed relieved. I'm sure he had no idea of what to do with me. This was before the Privacy Act, certainly before cell phones.

"We need to stop at my house to pick up your wallet for identification purposes and for your insurance information." There was a hospital nearby, but we drove to the far reaches of San Diego County because Mary knew that the local hospital there would take my insurance.

"How far are we going? It seems like we've been driving forever." My mind became clearer the longer we rode in the car. As we neared the hospital, I said "I feel better. I don't need a hospital."

"Well, we're going to the hospital regardless." Mary spoke firmly.

I joked around in the emergency room, wanting to believe nothing was wrong. I don't know what I thought was so funny. Maybe my head injury made me loopy. The doctor certainly didn't have a sense of humor and he didn't seem too sharp. He was tall, thin, and resembled a weasel. He hardly looked me over. "What about an X-ray?" I asked.

"You don't need one." He seemed annoyed that I asked. He couldn't do a CAT scan. They didn't exist until the early seventies and this was 1967. I was ready to leave the emergency room.

"Let's get out of here," I pleaded to Mary.

On the way back to Mary's house, I was hurting. In the ER, I had focused on my head, not my body. I should have been more serious with the doctor. I had landed first on my shoulder, then on my head. I had scraped my shoulder badly. Overall, I was pretty beaten up, more so than I first thought. I had a big bump and scrape on my head, and my right shoulder looked like minced meat. This all took place before wearing helmets had become the norm for bicyclists.

"You're going to go straight to bed," Mary insisted. "Your body has been traumatized so you must rest." I protested , but not hard. I ended up staying in bed or on the couch for a week.

That evening Mary pieced together what had happened. First, what I remember: We borrowed bikes from the minister at the La Jolla Presbyterian Church, who was friends with Mary and who had sons with bikes that I could borrow. Mary and I then rode around La Jolla so I could get a feel for the area. After a few hours we headed back to Mary's house which was in La Jolla Village at the bottom of a steep hill, when BAM! I went flying right over the handlebars. After that, all was a blank.

"I was ahead of you going down the hill," Mary said to me. "I thought you were behind me. When you didn't show up, I retraced my path."

When Mary put the mangled bike in the car, she noticed two bungee cords caught in the rear wheel. Apparently, the bungee cords slipped down and got caught in the spokes, causing the bike to come to a dead stop. "You were lucky you landed on your shoulder first and not on your head."

Why am I telling you this? Because this experience is my best guess as to why I have Parkinson's.

Fast forward to 1992, the year of my diagnosis. I wanted desperately to understand where this disease had come from. I repeatedly asked doctors, "Could there be a causal relationship between having a head injury and having Parkinson's?"

More than one neurologist answered, "There is no evidence of a connection." But fast forward another twenty years. Muhammad Ali's Parkinson's appears to have been caused from him constantly being pummeled by blows to the head. Football players are showing up with diagnoses of neurological damage because of all the head crushing they do while playing. And soldiers on the front line experience the worst head injuries of all.

"Couldn't Parkinson's be caused by a head injury?" I asked again years later. They are now researching this very question. I continue wondering.

I come from a large family with great longevity. My mother lived until she was just five months shy of a hundred years old. My grandmother lived until 98. Many of my relatives have lived or are living into their eighties or nineties. Heredity clearly did not cause my Parkinson's, as it does with some people. I am the only person in my family with it.

I never asked, "Why me?" Its corollary is, "Why not me?" If you ask one question, you have to ask the other. But my curiosity has always continued. Was it going to happen to me no matter what my life experiences presented? Is there anything I could have done to prevent it? Not ride a teenager's bike down a steep hill, I suppose.

Whether I simply pulled the short straw or had a head injury in my younger years, I probably will never know. I have come to terms with the proverbial saying, "It is what it is." Sometimes, that's all you can say.

Learning how to manage the "it is" has been my challenge. This mountain to climb has taken me on a journey in the second half of my life I never would have dreamed would be my path.

But, I'm still climbing.

Early Signs

"Change your thoughts and you change your world."
— *Norman Vincent Peale*

Looking back on "IT", as I do every day, I can see the signs. Taken individually, they seemed like non-events, but as I've reflected on them, I have to say, "Oh, that's what that was." Now it all adds up.

How about that lovely summer day on Squam Lake, at camp? My friend Jan and I were walking down the path to the waterfront. We were both councillors[1] at Singing Eagle Lodge, a girls' summer camp in New Hampshire, where we had met as campers more than forty years before. With her long legs, Jan literally bounced down the

---

[1] I am aware that the common spellings for this word are "counselor" and "councilor." Doc Ann, the founder of Singing Eagle Lodge in 1917 and its director until 1966, spelled the word with two "Ls," councillors. Old time campers and councillors still spell the word as Doc Ann did. The Thorndike-Barnhart Desk Dictionary, copyright 1951, states that "councillors" is the British spelling of the word.

steep path to the lake, except, of course, when she waited for me.

"Mopsy, does your arm bother you at all?"

"No, it's okay. It's fine," I replied casually, trying to hide my surprise by the concern in her voice. "What do you mean?"

"Well, you're holding your arm stiffly and it's not swinging when you walk. Looks like it hurts."

I didn't notice anything different and nothing hurt, so I dismissed her comment as that of an old friend aware that we were both getting older. Without each of us knowing it, Jan had just observed and given voice to my first sign that I was a Parkinsonian. A very heavy word.

A second sign that I ignored was from another camp friend, nicknamed Peach, who was my cabin roommate that summer. She laughingly said to me as we got dressed one morning, "Mopsy, you're a study in slow motion."

"That's not true," I replied. "I'm running on full throttle all the time."

"It may be," Peach said in her very direct voice, "but have you considered you're on the run because you're slow in getting started? It looks to me as though you're stuck in first gear. You're not going anywhere fast. Let's go to breakfast," Peach said. "I'll get you there on time."

We laughed all the way to the Wiggy, the dining hall at Singing Eagle Lodge.

Many of my friends called me "Grace" that summer because I was constantly tripping over roots on the paths, even though over many years, I had memorized where most of them were. I told my friends that I was just a first-class klutz that summer.

Back home, I enjoyed playing tennis with my son, and we would walk down the street to the high school courts to hit some balls. When I was his age, fifteen, I had played competitively and had won various local, club and camp tournaments.

One day after playing for a while, Stephen complained, "Mom, you aren't trying very hard today." I also had noticed that I wasn't playing well. My shots were really off and I could not get to the ball in time.

"I'm just tired, have a lot on my mind, and had a stressful morning," I replied. "I was hoping tennis would revive me." I could usually still beat Stephen despite his youth, but not that day.

My teenage daughter, Katie, was also on my case. "Mom, you always take a nap when you come home from work. You never used to do that."

"Well, I've been really busy at work and besides, I only lie down for about ten to fifteen minutes," I remarked, somewhat defensively. I, too, had noticed that I had been taking more naps, but hey, I was a single mom, working more than full time in a new career as an insurance agent, and raising two teenagers. Of course, I was tired.

When getting out of the car, I felt like an old lady. I had to push my way out of the driver's seat. With difficulty. Once upright, I would take a few very stiff steps, then walk the rest of the way to the door with little problem. I blamed my stiffness on possible arthritis. I convinced myself that *I was just fine.*

That year I spent the week after Christmas in Florida with my folks while my kids visited their dad. While working full time, I found I had no time earlier to write Christmas cards, so I gave myself permission to write them in the warmth of the Florida sun. It was important for me to write fairly long personal notes. Sending over one hundred holiday cards was my way of keeping in touch with friends from days past, from all over the country.

I discovered I needed a breather between each card I wrote. The first sentence or two were fairly legible. My handwriting grew steadily smaller and soon it was all a squiggly mess.

What was going on? Could it be a pinched nerve? Was it the hot Florida sun?

When I showed my handwriting to my mother, she said, "Martha, something IS going on. This is a far cry from your usual legible handwriting. Remember you had problems with your right arm after your surgery last summer to remove that ruptured appendix? Maybe it's related to that. You should check it out."

I was concerned, but I got those Christmas notes written and returned home with a tan.

Following up with the doctor to check what I thought was a pinched nerve was nowhere near the top of my "to-do" list. It took several more months before I got curious enough to check out my "pinched nerve."

Section 6

It Hasn't Gone Away...

Rotting Away

"Amidst the many thorns of living, there is always joy to be discovered, beauty to be seen, laughter to be heard, service to be accomplished, satisfaction to be found, love to be shared."
— *Scott Alexander*

Parkinson's disease eats away at me gradually. Being afflicted with Parkinson's is similar to any other process of slowly rotting away. Like an old tree stump, the odious part of the disease is progressing no matter how well I take care of myself. Like layers being pulled from an onion, my world becomes smaller and smaller.

The march of PD robs me of my independence, my strength, my ability to move, my ability to communicate. I measure the changes in my body by the things I can no longer do: walk without assistance, write legibly, drive my-self around town, get into and out of a car easily, turn a faucet, dress myself without a problem, or stand up from a chair, or couch. The list keeps growing.

After I bought my house on Chauncey Creek, I gave myself a month to get it ready before moving in. The walls needed painting so with the help of my daughter Katie, my brother Steve, and a variety of friends, we painted away. I enjoy painting. It isn't a chore. I would like to re-paint some walls now but I hate to envision the mess I would make if I picked up a paint brush today.

In the first few weeks of living in my new home, I hung a painting over the stairwell. This meant leaning over the second-floor railing, hammering in a nail, and then hang-ing a good-sized painting. I couldn't begin to do that now. In fact, today I can't even walk up the stairs by myself.

I once could flip my canoe into Chauncey Creek, pad-dle up the creek, return to the dock and flip it back onto the dock. A few years later I could get into a kayak or canoe only by flopping into it. I couldn't get out of the canoe without pulling up on something, often a person's leg. I gave my friends fits one day when I dumped my kayak over with me in it, figuring I could eject myself that way. I didn't win any prizes for that one. They yelled at me, "You scared us to death! Never do something that stupid again!" Now, some fifteen years later, I can't even walk to the dock without hanging on to somebody. Getting into a kayak or canoe can't be done.

I could garden when I first moved in; I took a perennial gardening class offered through adult ed. It was fun buying new plants and putting them in the ground. Now I have Kathy, who volunteers her time through the Master Gardener program to help take care of my garden. At this point I can do very little so I usually sit and talk with her, but I would rather be working next to her. She doesn't mind doing all the work. She worries that I might fall over the stone wall into the raspberry bushes.

The rotting of my body continues. I keep trying to counterattack it through exercise, spending time with friends, and trying to do the things I can no longer do or shouldn't be doing. It's so very frustrating not being able to do the things I used to do. I keep watching my layers peel away. It has been twenty-eight years and counting.

As I said earlier, I have never asked "Why me?" because I would have to ask its corollary, "Why not me?" I certainly have declined over the years. At times, I've felt discouraged, frustrated and worried about my future. "Why me?" has never been part of my vocabulary. But the jury is always out. One of these days I may very well yell: "Why me? What the fuck happened?"

Reality Check

"You gotta dance like there's nobody watching."
— *William W. Purkey*

"The first fifteen to twenty years were the easy ones. You're starting to deal with the tough ones, Martha," my neurologist proclaimed. Dr. Edward Drasby was a caring man, good with his patients, and he had a warm sense of humor, but that dreary day in November, he exhibited none of those qualities.

He explained that after twenty years with Parkinson's, medication was becoming less effective, with more side effects, and deep brain stimulation—DBS—wasn't going to rescue me anymore. DBS had saved me so far from dyskinesias, those writhing, gyrating, uncontrollable movements that I'd had such problems with before surgery. I remembered the neurologist at Johns Hopkins, where I'd had my surgery, telling me that deep brain stimulation wasn't a cure-all. But, I had always hoped that it would be. "DBS," he continued, "although wonderfully effective, doesn't deal with balance problems, the biggest problem with which you are dealing. So far, you've been lucky and haven't been hurt, particularly with the number of falls you've had."

I wanted to put a muzzle on him.

"People don't die from Parkinson's disease, but from its complications." He continued to explain that cracking my head on the corner of a cabinet or banging it on the floor can cause a serious brain bleed. That could kill me. Falling could cause broken bones. Aspirating food and liquids into my lungs could lead to pneumonia and even death.

I blinked. My body slumped. Enough for today.

Then there was Dayle, my homecare physical therapist, who arrived one day to give me physical therapy—and a good scolding—only weeks after Dr. Drasby had painted his dreadful picture. Dayle saw me twice a week and each time she reminded me to slow down and focus on moving my body forward so I wouldn't fall backward. She said that I tried to do too much.

Dayle, an attractive, sturdy looking woman, normally had a wonderful sense of humor, but that day she'd left it at home. Like Dr. Drasby, she wanted to set me straight. "You've got to accept that you aren't going to get better,

Martha. You have Parkinson's disease. There is a spot, deep in your brain, that is screwed up—the substantia nigra."

Dr. Drasby and Dayle desperately wanted me to stay upright and not injure myself. They couldn't have been more direct—or more serious. It was hard to hear that my problems were progressing, that I would never get better, even though I knew it to be true. The reality of their saying so was jarring.

Even the general public is trying to get me to slow down. I have to ask myself, *why don't I slow down?* I have taken many falls, but only one was caused by my walking with a walker. The vast majority of my falls have taken place while I'm standing. They happen when I'm focused on something other than what my body is doing.

As I was leaving a local restaurant with my walker, I passed by a table near the door and heard a woman say, "Slow down. You're going too fast." I laughed and told her she should see me when I'm fired up.

At a shoe store, I was trying to find some shoes to wear with the brace on my right foot. Making a few laps around the store, trying on different shoes, the woman waiting on me said in an astonished voice, "I can't believe how fast you move in that walker. Don't go fast on my account. I'm here all day."

My friend, Lynn, used to say, "Martha is hopeless. She's faster than a lot of us."

I knew I was never going to climb Mt. Washington again as I did in the earlier stages of my disease. My reality and struggle now involved climbing Mount Parkinson.

In my earlier years of hiking, when I reached the summit of any mountain, I felt accomplished and fulfilled. The view was always glorious. But, as I climb Mount Parkinson's, I know I'll never conquer it. The bar keeps moving. It isn't a fun climb. And it gets tougher each year. That's because there's no end in sight, except the ultimate one when, as my father said, "You check out for good."

I must adjust. I can't return to who I was, but I want to. I'm tired of adapting. I want to walk with my friends, play tennis and golf, paddle a canoe, climb a mountain, hold my grandchildren. Becoming more debilitated scares me. But most of all, I want to stay alive. I am not ready to check out yet.

Frustrations

"Resting is not laziness, it's medicine!"
— Glenn Schweitzer

People who don't have Parkinson's or who don't live with someone who does, have no idea what it takes to get through the day. It's a challenge from morning till night. Getting out of bed and getting dressed used to be easy before Parkinson's reared its ugly head. Then it became a chore. And now, I need a twenty-four-hour caregiver.

I've had to learn that "nothing" is actually a new "something." I used to walk three days a week, swim two days, stretch and do Tai Chi—all things to stay healthy. (Yeah, a nap got thrown in here and there, too.) Now, all that is just a dim memory. Yet here I still am, still talking (or writing) to all of you. But I admit, despite fighting and surviving this dreadful condition for twenty-eight years ... and counting, I still haven't adjusted to the new me.

The new me doesn't win prizes for speed. Now, I use an electronic wheelchair, bumping around all over the house, crashing into furniture and walls and sometimes taking the radiator covers right off. I usually laugh if someone is with me because I can't believe what I am doing. I also have trouble eating without spilling, cutting my food and holding onto my utensils, piles of papers and anything else in my hands.

I used to love using a pen to write, but I had to turn to this computer when I could no longer read my own handwriting. So, here I sit, punching keys.

Right now, I'm really frustrated, sitting here in front of my computer, trying to type this vignette. My fingers keep hitting a key next to the one I want. I'm making spaces in words that shouldn't be there. Often, I can't remember what word I meant to write in the first place. I'm still part of my weekly writing group although I can't comment on somebody else's work as quickly as I used to, and when I do speak up, people can't hear me or understand me. But my fellow writers encourage me to show up, and I do.

Friends have helped me tremendously, driving me places, but I got to the point where I had too much difficulty getting in and out of a car. The advantage of having a 24/7 caregiver is that now I always have someone who can give me a ride and I can go where I want to.

When I'm in a public space, maybe sitting in my wheelchair during intermission at a concert, I'm surrounded by my friends, chatting away. But their conversations are taking place above me. I would love to join them, but even if I could stand, my voice has gotten so soft and low, it's tough for me to talk and for them to hear me. Maybe I should start a belly button club. That's where I am. That's all I see.

I used to be able to wear nice sweaters and shirts with buttons but now it's only over-your-head shirts because it's gotten too hard for me—or my helper—to put them on. I'm thinking I should join a nudist colony so clothes wouldn't be an issue, but it gets cold up here in Maine.

Sleeping is hard work, too. I used to be the 'put your head on the pillow' type who doesn't move till morning. And right now, I'm really tired, PD tired. I haven't slept all night in years. So here I sit, punching my keys, in this, my twenty-eighth year with IT. I sometimes think I'm better off than I am, and sometimes I know I'm worse off than others think. I've got us all fooled.

Festinations

Life is a question and how we live it is our answer.
— Gary Keller

Hearing me clumping up her sidewalk with my walker, Bonnie came running down her porch steps to greet me. Old college friends, we'd lived on opposite coasts until recently. We hadn't seen each other in more than ten years. But here I was, visiting with my twenty-plus years of PD. I continued bumping toward her in the bright July sun, eager to connect, when my body came to a dead stop, stiffening so abruptly I nearly fell over my walker. "I'm freezing," I gasped. "I'm freezing."

Bonnie shot toward me, her arms stretched out in a hug. Just as quickly, she released her hold on my suddenly rigid body and shouted, "Don't worry, Mopsy. Stay right there! I'll be right back." What else did she think I could do? I remained helpless, watching her racing back up to the house, her blond hair flying behind her.

She was back immediately, a blue navy sweater in her hand. "What's this?" I asked, my body just as suddenly back in my control.

"This sweater's for you, silly," she said, as she helped me up her steps. "I knew something was wrong when you said you were freezing. In July? In New England with all its hot and humid weather? I knew it had to be that crazy disease of yours, throwing you another curve ball."

"You're right," I said as we made our way into her house. "My 'freezing' has nothing to do with being cold. It's this confounded disease, and it's really frightening because I never know when another episode is going to happen. And there's absolutely nothing I can do about it."

"My pot of coffee is all set," Bonnie said, "but I first need you to admire my wonderful oak table that I recently inherited from my mother. I sat at it every night growing up and we're going to sit at it right now. Let's raise our coffee cups to my mother. I know she would have been thrilled to know that we're together."

Sitting down at her special oak table, all I wanted to do was to talk to my old friend, to share my fears, and a few of the frustrations that often threatened to overwhelm me. "It's called 'festination,'" I muttered. "Festination," I said again, spitting out the word as if it were a rotten piece of fruit.

"Sure sounds dirty to me," Bonnie said with a wry smile as she pushed a plate of raspberry scones toward me.

"Yeah, it's a new PD thing," I said. "My body just stops dead until it decides to move again. I don't decide, and I can't stop it from happening. And if I don't go rigid or just get stuck in a doorway, this quirky thing makes me take tiny little steps," I said, rushing on, glad to be sharing with my old friend. "But then I start going so fast I lose my balance and crash to the floor."

"That sure doesn't sound good," Bonnie said, bringing her chair and our coffee cups closer.

"Maybe I'll buy a laser pointer," I said, "you know, the kind business people use for presentations. I hear that drawing a red line with the pointer somehow breaks the spell, and we PD'ers can move again. That'll be one of my new tricks."

Pressing my hand, Bonnie looked at me intently, her voice low. "You've fought this awful thing for so long, Mopsy. What is it that has kept you going?" Sitting there with my old friend, her hand in mine, we both knew the answer was here, having support like this.

Northeast Rehab

"You either get bitter or you get better. It's that simple. You either take what has been dealt to you and allow it to make you a better person, or you allow it to tear you down. The choice does not belong to fate, it belongs to you."

— *Josh Ship*

How did I get so lucky?

I was beginning my third decade with Parkinson's disease, increasingly hopeless about this disorder ravaging my body. I was envious of those new programs for Parkinson patients I was always reading about that were happening in places like Boston, New York and San Francisco.

But I lived on the Maine seacoast—the place where I had finally found my dream house right on the water. I could still make my way out to the deck each morning and enjoy the gulls circling, but it was getting harder and harder to get through the rest of the day.

Then along came Lisa Sommers. Speaking to our York County Parkinson's support group one afternoon, this short, attractive woman talked about her passion for starting a Parkinson's facility with programs offering different therapies—with programs for yoga, general exercise, boxing and LSVT training (Lee Silverman Voice Technique) designed specifically for Parkinson's patients.

One year later, it happened, serving the entire seacoast area of New Hampshire and of southern Maine, the opening of the Outpatient Unit at Northeast Rehabilitation Hospital. I was there the first week and have been a fixture ever since.

It was immediately clear that the therapists who greeted me each week had skilled knowledge about all kinds of neurological disorders. It was also clear their primary focus would be Parkinson's disease and that I would be a primary beneficiary of programs specifically designed for Parkinson's.

Julie and Dave, physical therapists who specialized in Parkinson's. Laurie, occupational therapist. Lisa, speech therapist, and now Terri, another speech therapist who filled Lisa's spot as she moved on to be the head of the master's program in speech therapy at U Mass Amherst.

These rehab therapists have impressed me for their dedication and skilled knowledge about patients with neurological disorders. At least at the beginning, they have primarily focused on Parkinson's disease. They are extremely challenging to patients and treat us with kindness and sense of humor, a bonus.

Sarah, the receptionist with dark hair, glasses, and usually wearing a cardigan sweater, is the first person you see as you come into the building. She's always ready for a quick conversation and a good laugh.

The reception area is a large, open and attractive space with comfortable couches and chairs. A huge stone fireplace stretches to the ceiling, which is at least two stories high. It is a space that is very inviting. Many friendships have been forged here, I believe, because the ambience of the room encourages engagement with others. It's a happy place, particularly for those who look like we do with trembling hands, who walk very stiffly and have great difficulty getting out of a chair or a couch.

Carole sits next to Sarah at the reception desk. She often says to me, "Martha, I'll never forget you." She goes on to say that I was one of the first patients to sign up for their LSVT Big and Loud program, the first program held for Parkinson's patients in the Seacoast area of New Hampshire and Southern Maine.

Carole reminds me that at the very first day of registration for the new outpatient clinic, she left the room for a brief moment to get a form. During that time I fell to the floor. When she ran back into the room, I was on the floor, laughing.

She recalls the terror she felt as she went to help me up. "But you were just like a clown on a trampoline. You just bounced back up and with a smile on your face, said, 'Bet you didn't expect that, did you?' "

Since that first day, I have been one of their favorite and most loyal customers.

Boxing

"It's not about how hard you can hit; it's about how hard you can get hit and keep moving forward."
— *Rocky Balboa*

"Take that ... that, and ... THAT! Parkinson's, you are not welcome in my life." *WHAP, WHAP, WHAP!* Dave, our instructor, had propped a thick red exercise mat upright at the end of the room. He instructed us to take turns hitting the mat hard for thirty seconds at a time. I volunteered to go first. As I hit the red mat, all I started to see was red. I found myself yelling at the mat, and the louder I yelled, the harder and faster I hit.

"Parkinson's, you have robbed me of so much. GO AWAY!" The others in the group cheered me on. Thirty seconds seems like such a minuscule amount of time, but each turn I took hitting the mat was intense physically, and mentally also very, very satisfying.

We were a disparate crew of eight, experiencing our symptoms differently, and in various stages of disability, all participating in Boxing for Parkinson's. That's right, Boxing for Parkinson's. The classes were offered to improve our balance.

Though Dave had started these wonderful classes for Parkinson's, he doesn't look much like a boxer. He's tall and lanky, has a somewhat bald head, always has a wide smile, and is genuinely a nice person.

In order to be in the group, three of us needed to be tethered to individual staff members. They stood behind each of us holding onto our belts so we wouldn't fall, and giving us many words of encouragement. We took turns throwing punches at Dave for about thirty minutes, then came ten minutes of kickboxing.

We started each session just like the professional boxers do. Dave or his assistants wrapped straps about an inch wide around both of our hands. The straps were flexible enough to intertwine between fingers, and long enough to wrap around our fingers and hands at least three times. Next, on went the gloves. At first, I was surprised the gloves were so stiff and had no flexibility to them. At least they were red.

After wrapping our hands, we started by standing in a circle doing some arm exercises to warm up. Then Dave put on a pair of mitts that were flat with a target in the middle of each one. We took turns trying to hit the targets on his mitts with the punches we'd learned, whether with crosscuts, a jab, or one of the other various punches. With each punch we shifted our weight from the right foot to the left.

We took turns kickboxing, following Dave as he worked his way across the room. Jabs and cross jabs, kicks against a target more than a foot off the ground. At first, I was amazed that I could do this at all, let alone without falling. It's been four years now but I'm still boxing—if only in my dreams.

Shortly after I started boxing class at the age of 73, I was listening to a call-in radio show. A woman, aged 60, described herself as a senior citizen. A few days later I read an article in the paper about an "elderly" woman in a car crash. She was 72.

I've never considered myself a senior citizen, nor did I consider myself elderly at 73.

Section 7

Experiences Along the Way

Climbing Mt. Washington

"I have found that if you love life,
it will love you back."
— *Arthur Rubenstein*

"We're going to get you up there one more time." This was my friend Amy around three years after my Parkinson's diagnosis, about joining her climb to New England's highest peak east of the Mississippi.

At lunchtime Amy walked into the dining hall at Singing Eagle Lodge with the group of campers she had just led up Mt. Washington. She was wearing a pink T-shirt that boasted, "This body climbed Mt. Washington." I had bought that T-shirt a number of years before as a councillor at Singing Eagle Lodge, the girl's camp I was a part of on Squam Lake in the White Mountains of New Hampshire. The shirt was passed down from year to year to the councillor in charge of the Mt. Washington climb. She took off the shirt and gave it to me. The shirt had come full circle.

I had climbed Mt. Washington and the Presidential Range three or more times as a camper and twice as a councillor. The climb was not a casual one. Mt. Washington is, yes, New England's highest peak east of the Mississippi, a little more than one mile high. Its summit experienced the fastest wind speed ever recorded—231 MPH— until its record was broken in 2010 on Barrow Island in Australia with a wind speed of 253 MPH.

Mt. Washington is known for its erratic and quickly deteriorating weather. It offers climbers the dire warning:

<u>STOP</u>

THIS AREA HAS THE WORST WEATHER IN AMERICA.

MANY HAVE DIED FROM EXPOSURE EVEN IN THE SUMMER.

TURN BACK NOW IF THE WEATHER IS BAD.

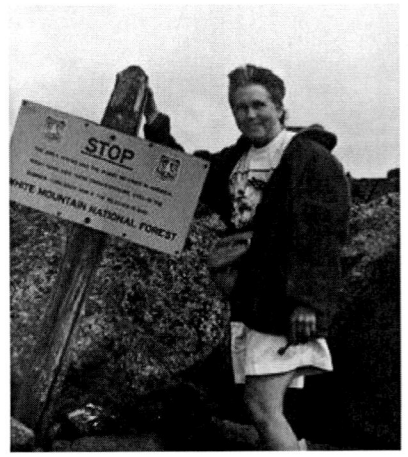

Now, three years into living with Parkinson's, Amy was encouraging me to climb Mt. Washington again and found a group of friends who wanted to climb it with us. We were seven strong—Amy, Jesse, Susie, Jill, Linda, Laura, and me. Five of us had known each other since summer camp days when we were eleven or twelve years old. We were now in our fifties and our friendship was as solid as New Hampshire granite. Jesse and Amy were half our ages. Their friendship was just as valued.

"We're going to get you up there one more time." Those challenging words were repeated.

I knew it was a three-day hike and a difficult climb. My body had changed and was continuing to change. It was deteriorating, just like Mt. Washington's weather.

I had climbed it before but never as someone with Parkinson's disease. To get ready for this climb I had been working out at the gym and swimming regularly.

DAY ONE

On a beautiful July day in 1995 our mighty crew of longtime friends gathered at the starting point of the Ammonoosuc Trail at the base of Mt. Washington, I with my Leki hiking poles in hand. I had bought them specifically for this climb. My friends kindly divvied up the items in my backpack to lighten my load and we took off. Each of us felt excited about the climb ahead.

The beginning of the trail was fairly easy. Then it suddenly took a right-angled turn. Upward. From then on it was a challenge. A tough challenge. My poles got me over the streams without taking a dunk. They gave me much-needed support and balance. At times it was close. I weaved back and forth while trying to get to the other side on more than one slippery log.

Was I going to make it?

At times I wondered. My friends helped me up the vertical ladders that were attached to the side of the mountain. Our biggest obstacle was laughter. We all felt the process was hilarious. One or two friends got below me and pushed. Two others would kneel above me, pulling me up by my belt loops. They managed to swing my legs up when I couldn't swing them up on my own.

The longer we climbed, the shorter the trees became, until we were surrounded only by scrub pine. At one point, we had to cross a steep, bald and very large rock face. I tripped, fell to my knees, and then lied flat.

"I'm going to slide right off the mountain," I said with trepidation in my voice.

"No, you're doing fine. Just keep moving towards us," came reassuring voices.

"Are you sure I'm not going to slide down the mountain?"

"No, we wouldn't let you do that. Here, hold onto this scrub pine. It's sturdy. It's not going to get ripped out while you pull on it."

I remembered looking up after we had been hiking for three hours and after my ordeal with the rock face.

THE LAKE OF THE CLOUDS!

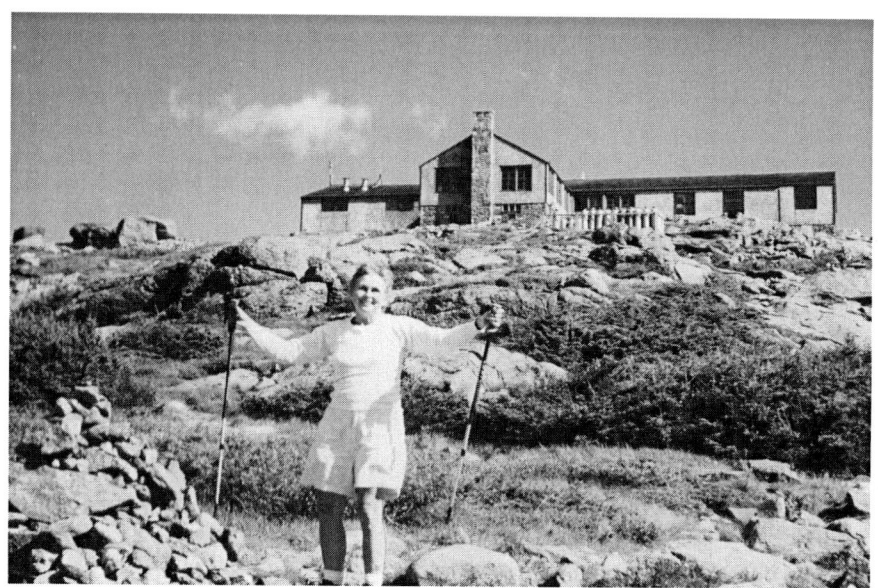

I had made it to the lake and the hut, our sleeping spot for the next two nights. I laughed with relief. Climbing to the Lake of the Clouds hut completed the most difficult part of the trip. I knew the summit was only two hours beyond and was something that we would tackle in the morning. I raised my poles in thanksgiving.

At the hut, we were greeted by three of our group who had gone ahead earlier when I needed to slow down. The group who made it up first warned us that we were to share our bunk room with eight or nine campers from a boy's camp in northern New Hampshire. They were fourteen and fifteen years old. They must have seen us as relics from the past.

After getting organized, we went outside to soak up the sunshine. We each found rock formations into which we could nestle our bodies. I fell fast asleep.

Before dinner we searched the bookshelves for the musty, old logbooks from the late '50s to the early '60s. Each summer, fresh log books were made available for climbers to sign their names and make comments. Nostalgia set in when I found one of the logbooks I had signed with my youthful—and readable—handwriting in 1959.

After a well prepared and quite tasty family style turkey dinner, the AMC (Appalachian Mountain Club) staff, most of whom were college students, put on a skit for us. They used the skit to remind us that the food and supplies had to be backpacked in two or three times a week. Each pack of food weighed about ninety pounds.

After the skit, we prepared ourselves for bed. In the bathroom, there was a step up of about a foot into the toilet stall area. I was holding onto the door handle for support, about to take the step up when the door unexpectedly swung wide open. I had leaned too hard on it. I flew to the other side of the room, directly into a solid, cement wall.

"OH, SHIT!"

Amy ran for an AMC volunteer and brought back two bags of frozen peas and a concerned AMC worker. She advised me, "Keep these bags of peas on your head since you have quite a lump." Amy stayed with me as the hut lights were turned out for the night. We eventually made it to bed with flashlights to light the way.

DAY TWO

We awoke to the clanging of a metal spoon against an aluminum pot. We didn't exactly jump out of bed. We let the boys get a head start so we could have a little more privacy.

Breakfast was hardy and I was starved. Oatmeal, scrambled eggs, toast, coffee, and juice. The AMC worker bees instructed us on how to shake out and fold the blankets we had used the night before. They had to be folded just so, and then placed at the foot of the bed for the next people coming through. I wondered when the blankets were cleaned and who carried them up and down the mountain.

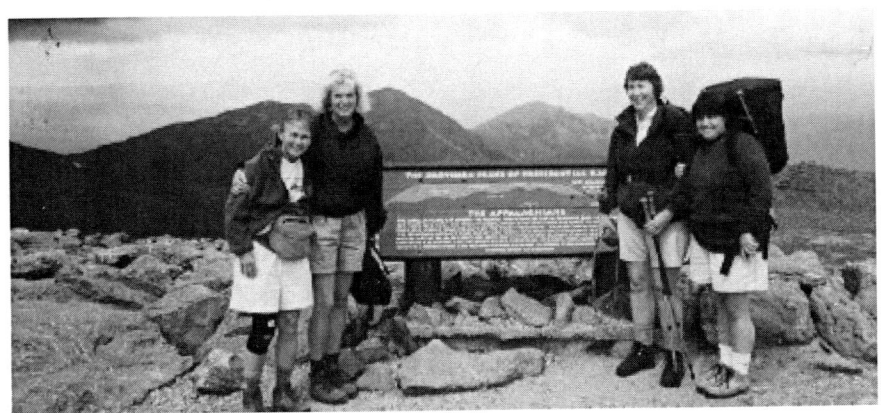

Myself, Jill Wickes Burrill, Susan Kemp, and Laura Livingston.

We added sandwiches, snacks and water to our packs and headed off. Not too far from the hut we came to the sign warning us that weather on Mt. Washington could deteriorate quickly. Fortunately, we had no signs of impending bad weather and, instead, had a glorious day ahead of us.

Around the Lake of the Clouds hut were colorful wildflowers and occasional groups of scrub pine, but soon the path gave way to boulders. The views were spectacular because the weather was clear. I remember as a camper on one of our trips climbing in nothing but fog. This time we were blessed with sunshine all three days on the mountain. I preferred this.

I was the last one to reach the top of Mt. Washington along with one of my friends determined to stay with me. Hugs were freely given and received. We had made it. A ticker tape parade would have been no more satisfying. We found the sign at the summit that said very simply:

MT. WASHINGTON SUMMIT
ELEV. 6288 FEET

A kind gentleman volunteered to take our picture as we gathered around the sign. He was interested in our story.

We saw the building there that allowed us to buy and mail postcards, along with T-shirts and trinkets. I had been seeing a therapist at the time and I remembered when she asked, "Have you thought about if you don't make it?" I responded with confidence, "That is not an option. I'm going to send you a postcard from the top." Which I did.

After a few hours at the top, we headed down to the hut. So often it's easier to climb up than to go down. That was our case. The danger was moving too fast, losing your footing, and not being able to stop. We found ourselves jumping from one boulder to another.

"Mopsy, please don't jump over a crevasse or at least warn us before you do. You're going to give us all heart attacks."

I had not yet accepted my limitations. I still have difficulty with that, all these years later.

———//———

DAY THREE

On the third day we had two options to get down the mountain: climb down the way we came or climb back up to the summit and take the cog railway down. Four in the group chose to climb down and three of us climbed to the top to ride the railway.

I didn't care how I got down. I had accomplished what I had come to accomplish. Getting up the mountain.

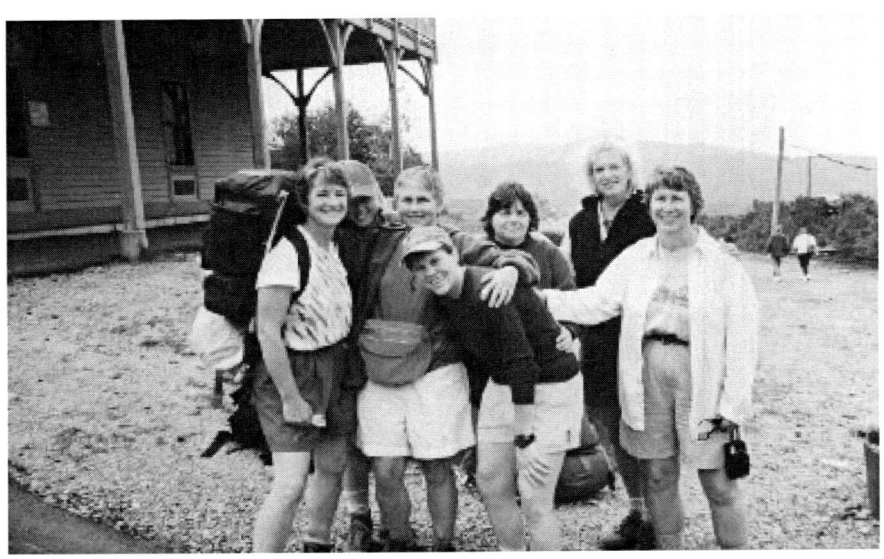

Back at the bottom.

Gifts from Africa

"I have no choice about whether or not I have Parkinson's. I have nothing but choices about how I react to it. In those choices, there's freedom to do a lot of things in areas I wouldn't have otherwise found myself in."

— Michael J. Fox

During a ten-hour or so plane ride, we woke to the sound of whirring engines, looked out the window and saw sand. Lots of sand. "That's the Sahara Desert down there," I exclaimed. My friend Ellie and I were on our way to Kenya and Tanzania. Ellie with her reddish hair, tiny body and wonderful sense of humor. Me, in my early years of Parkinson's, my neck stiff and my knees weak. Fortunately, we laugh a lot when we are together.

When Ellie and Rick invited me for dinner a few months after their wedding, the topic of Africa came up, so Rick pulled out his slides of climbing Kilimanjaro and going on a safari. Ellie and I oohed and aahed. "If you want to go to Africa, you should go." I looked at Rick as he sat in his wheelchair. Knowing that he wouldn't be able to go on a safari again made me realize that, if I wanted to go, I couldn't wait. If I had waited, I never would have gone. Rick said, "Start planning your trip now." We did.

It took a touch of craziness for me to go, particularly when I considered the financial ramifications. Although I had two kids in college at the time, I knew there was no better time to go than now. I'd had my Parkinson's diagnosis for four years and I knew I had to do things before Parkinson's totally took over my body.

All three of us were keenly aware that anything could happen to anyone at any time. I had Parkinson's, and Rick had become a paraplegic after flying in a helicopter that crashed while working as a civil engineer in Alaska. Rick was incredibly grateful he had traveled as much as he had before the accident, and Ellie was just as aware as we were that anyone's life can change in an instant.

In Kenya we learned a Swahili word, "pole-pole" [pronounced pole-ee, pole-ee], which translates to "slowly-slowly." Having less energy and being slower, I identified all too well with that phrase. Ellie teased me and said laughingly, "Keep up, Martha." I replied I was enjoying the pole-pole time and learning patience, and she'd just have to wait.

The drivers on our game drives taught us lots about practicing patience. To learn about animal behavior and if we wanted to see animals, we had to appreciate the importance of quietly and patiently waiting. As a result, we had incredible animal sightings.

"Look at those lions playing so joyfully, rolling in the dirt, jumping on each other's backs and chasing each other around," Ellie said one morning. We giggled at the antics of the cubs. 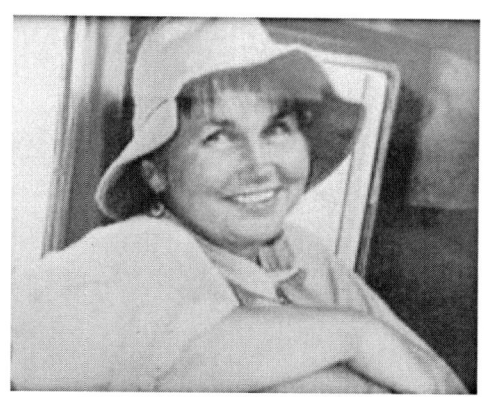 Ellie had told me many times that if she only saw one animal on this trip, it would have to be a lion. We saw lions mating. One fellow with its sexy mane let out a huge roar as he and his lioness enjoyed each other. No privacy for them. There they were, in the wild.

We saw giraffes ambling regally across the landscape —so much taller and freer than giraffes in our zoos. Why did I like the giraffes so much? I didn't identify with them at all. I've never been called regal or graceful in my life, and I certainly don't have a neck that moves so easily. Perhaps I favored them because I knew their grace was something to which I could never aspire.

The elephants were as huge as I had imagined, traveling as families while nuzzling their adorable babies along the way. Hippos in the "hippo pools" produced a chorus of every bodily sound imaginable. And I imagined the hippos and the elephants all greeting me and saying, "Hi, Mopsy. So glad you visited us. We move slowly here, too, just as you do."

The leopards seemed to spend their days sleeping on the tree limbs, their paws and tales dangling, before getting up to stretch, turn around and flop back down. On our last morning as we left the crater, a leopard crossed the bumpy dirt road directly in front of our van, went into the bushes next to us and stopped to stare at us eyeball to eyeball, a mere six feet away. Our hearts stopped. I was grateful to have the window glass between us.

Our greatest lesson about patience and trust came at the end of our last and very long day in the Ngorongoro Crater, our last full day on safari. Ellie and I were dusty, tired, and ready to call it a day, to head up to our lodge on the rim of the crater for a quick "lie-down" leopard style, shower, and glass of wine with dinner.

But, Martin, our native driver, had other ideas. He stopped our Land Rover, climbed out the opening in the roof, and pointed to a black speck in the distance. "It's a black rhino," he whispered. "We must wait for it to get closer." Ellie and I rolled our eyes. We could barely see the black dot with our binoculars but we trusted Martin. The intenseness of his eyes made us believers.

But the black speck stayed that way for what felt like an eternity. We continued to wait because our guts told us that we were going to witness something incredible. Martin next inched the Land Rover slowly along the crater wall. Climbing to the roof for another look through his

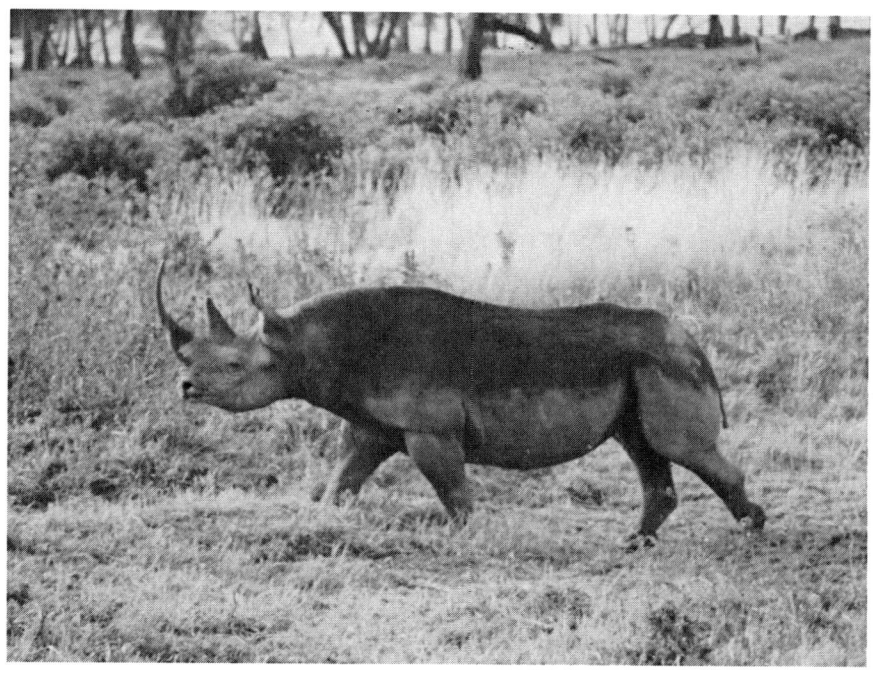

binoculars, he exclaimed, "It's moving! It's moving towards us!" We could see nothing, but we knew to trust Martin's instincts. His eyes were riveting.

Martin had claimed just a few moments earlier, if we were going to see the rhino up close, the rhino had to pass through what was a long line of migrating wildebeest. They looked like unshaven buffalo. Spotting us more clearly, the rhino came more quickly, making a few stops to check if we were still there.

About fifty feet away, he stopped and stared directly at our van. A rhino is a massive animal, and he was not smiling. We sucked in some air and held our breath. We knew rhinos could charge vans, even trains. This was for real. It was the first time on the trip that I felt fear.

We started breathing again as the rhino walked closer to our Land Rover. About thirty feet away, he stopped twice to spray and mark his territory, then slowly moved in front of us, stopped, started again, moved right along- side our van, then disappeared into the woods.

Because we were willing to be patient, we had been able to witness a tiny, black speck in the distance become a huge black rhino staring at us. A treasured experience. What it took on our part was trust and patience. And for me, the determination to live my life with all its possibilities for as long as I could.

I thought about Rick as he sat in his wheelchair back home. I took a deep breath considering all the challenges he had met and was continuing to meet. I knew that Parkinson's would present me with many more challenges as my condition progressed, but I as I think back over the last twenty or so years, I'm so glad that I had said, "YES, YES to Africa!"

Parkinson's Unity Walk

*Never let the things you cannot do prevent you
from doing the things you can."*
— Coach John Wooden

The call came out of nowhere. "Mom, are you sitting down?" Katie didn't wait for my answer. "We're going to go to New York City, in April" she said, her voice happy, excited. "I've signed us up to join the Parkinson's Unity Walk in Central Park this year."

"Oh? How did this come about?" I replied, so stunned I could barely speak. Ever since I had told my kids my devastating news nine years earlier Katie had barely mentioned Parkinson's to me. And I was sure she hadn't told any of her friends.

"I noticed all kinds of groups have walks to raise money for their particular cause, but I had never heard of such a walk or run to benefit Parkinson's research. So, I went

148

online, and I discovered there's a Parkinson's Unity Walk every April in Central Park. One hundred percent of the funds raised each year are designated for Parkinson's research, and I liked that. So, I signed us up."

And just like that, Team Mopsy was born.

Team Mopsy has participated in the Unity Walk every year since 2004. What is so rewarding is the support we've received both from people who want to participate in the walk and those who contribute so generously to the cause. The bulk of the fundraising has been Katie's doing. The first year, Katie set an initial goal of $2500, then increased her pledge fairly quickly to $5000 and ended up raising a little less than $10,000. Overall, Team Mopsy has donated more than $170,000 for Parkinson's research—and counting. Katie has been one of the top twenty fundraisers almost every year since we started participating.

Katie's method of fundraising has worked well for her. She first came up with a list of friends and acquaintances with whom she felt comfortable asking for money. I did the same. She then wrote letters to potential donors, explaining my situation, talking about the walk, and asking for a donation.

"Mom, I'm amazed how people are responding,"

Katie said. "People I hardly know are sending in checks, donating to the cause."

What meant so much to people was that Katie wrote handwritten thank you notes to each person who donated. "Your Katie is something," friends would say to me. "Her notes mean so much."

Katie brought along some college friends that first year at the walk and they've come back almost every year. And, she's added some other friends along the way, as have I. The group has swelled.

My long-time camp friends were there from the start. At the end of the first walk, I was very touched by their enthusiasm, but figured it would be a one-time deal for them.

"No way," they all chimed in. "We're in this for the long haul." I made these "forever friends" at Singing Eagle Lodge. Each of us has known each other for more than fifty years. They haven't missed a year in supporting Katie and me.

I was especially happy when my son Stephen and his wife Arabella and their two boys joined us. Luke was a one-year-old, and Alex only eighteen months older. Now they bring along three, with Anna making her debut a few years later. Their "Team Mopsy" T-shirts came down to their ankles at first but they have since grown into them. I love catching first sight of them as they come running, arms outstretched, yelling, "Hi, Gami! We love you!"

The walk the first year was emotionally overwhelming. Watching the long line of Parkinsonians wending their way through the park, however slowly, with their families and friends was immensely moving. The day was nothing short of perfect.

I felt joy and sadness all wrapped into one. Joy at seeing so many people together dealing with the same illness, including the well-known Janet Reno, Attorney General under President Clinton, and actor and activist Michael J. Fox, who spoke to the people before the walk began and then joined the walkers.

"We all want the same thing," said Michael J. Fox. "A cure for Parkinson's."

SERENDIPITY MOMENTS

"Let's go find Mopsy in New York City today. It's a gorgeous sunny, blue-sky day. Mopsy, her kids and grandkids, and a variety of friends will be in Central Park with her for the Unity Walk."

Sky responded to Melinda, saying, "I'm all set to go." Pomfret, Connecticut, where they lived, wasn't exactly around the corner from the city. It was at least a two-hour drive for them, but they both were up for it.

Melinda said that when they first arrived at the park, they were overwhelmed by the throngs of people. "How are we ever going to find Mopsy with all these people?" Both Melinda and Sky were wondering the same thing at the same time. But since they'd made the journey, they decided they might as well start walking.

Miraculously they found me within five minutes. I felt a tap on my shoulder. As I turned to look behind me, Melinda swung around in front of me.

"MELINDA!" I screeched. We stood in the middle of the path we were on and hugged each other as other walkers streamed around us.

Two years later I was at another Unity Walk, along with 10,000 other people, when I heard a voice ask, "Is that you, Martha?" I have known very few Marthas in this world. I looked up in spite of that, never guessing that someone was calling out for me. I was dead wrong.

As I looked around I saw Lisa Sommers making her way—sideways—across a long line of people who were wending their way along the Parkinson's route.

Lisa had taken a new position as a clinical graduate

professor at U Mass Amherst, having left her position as speech pathologist at Northeast Rehab where I'd gotten to know her. It didn't surprise me that she'd brought along five or six grad students to the Unity Walk, thinking of her strong commitment to Parkinson's.

Yet another year, I heard voices screaming, "Team Mopsy! Team Mopsy!" It was my dear friend Marcia Gibbons, who was in New York with her daughter and three nieces to celebrate a birthday. They were perched on the back of one of the benches, visible and loud. I had just seen Marcia yesterday at home in Kittery Point, not even twelve hours earlier.

That I call serendipity.

It's Heaven

"Life keeps throwing me stones. And I keep finding diamonds."
— Ana Claudia Antunes

She bounces in the door every Wednesday afternoon at four-thirty, with bag in hand, a smile on her face, and a cheery "Hello, Martha," in her lilting South African voice. "I'm late again."

"Don't worry about it. You walk to my house every Wednesday, faithfully, regardless of the weather. You're like the post office, come rain or shine. Besides, I'm not a paying customer." We hug and head to the sunroom where we delight in each other's company. In the summer, it's the deck overlooking Chauncey Creek.

Bridgit lives four houses down the creek from me. We have known each other for more than twenty years now. We have much in common: born the same year, bought our houses within a year of each other, both with the same mortgage agent who introduced us. We each have two grown children, successful in their own rights. We love the outdoors and both of us are grateful each day for living on Chauncey Creek. Bridgit is an acupuncturist by profession, a fun-loving woman who, just by chance, loves to massage feet.

"Oh, I forgot to get us some water." As I attempt to move forward in my chair to get up, Bridgit jumps up and flies into the kitchen. "You sit tight. You aren't supposed to do anything during this hour except relax."

As Bridgit returns with the water, I start taking my shoes off. "Here, give me your feet." She takes off my shoes, socks, and the leg brace that I wear to help keep my right foot straight, puts a towel over the ottoman, pulls the apricot kernel oil from her bag, and starts massaging my feet.

Bridgit takes my right foot first because that's the foot that has both arthritis and Parkinson's. Her hands are gentle and strong.

Bliss.

I confess to her that I am embarrassed by my feet being not particularly beautiful. My big toes usually have marks on them. They tend to curl up which causes my shoes to rub on my toes. Once again Parkinson's rears its ugly head, this time with dystonia—abnormal muscle tone. I cramp up a lot.

My cell phone timer goes off exactly at five-thirty p.m. It alerts me to take the evening dose of my Parkinson's medication. "I hate having to interrupt us, but I'm lucky to have that timer to remind me to take my drugs. Cell phones do have some redeeming features after all." We laugh. Bridgit knows how I feel about all those electronic gadgets that surround us. While I take my pills, she sits back, sighs, and drinks some water.

We talk about everything for that hour we are together. We laugh a lot, and talk about the books we've read, the movies we've seen, recipes worth sharing, the affairs of the world. We often boast that if the "higher-ups" would only listen to us, the world would be a better place. Bridgit talks about growing up in Cape Town, South Africa, at a time when apartheid was still in place. A lot of tension. She recalls having certain books that had to be kept under cover or they could be confiscated. Scary times.

Our kids and grandkids don't get left out of the conversation. They're often central to it. Bridgit has twelve grandchildren, ten of whom are from one family. The two others are granddaughter twins. "Whew," I say, "how do you do it?"

"Not easy," she says, "not easy." But Bridgit is up to the task. "Keeping up with birthdays is the hardest."

I regale her with the antics of my three grandchildren, Alex, Luke, and Anna. A lot of funny stories are exchanged. I remember one in particular, telling her about the day a few years earlier when Anna, then three, followed me into the sun room, where I normally put my shoes on. As I reached for my brace, she asked, "Gami, can I help you?"

"Of course, I'd love your help."

The first step was putting on my socks. I helped her do that, then I watched with astonishment as she put the brace on my right foot and then tightened the two velcro straps. She even picked out the right shoe for the right foot and the left shoe for the left foot. Amazing—at three years of age!

The hour is up. Bridgit packs up and insists on putting my foot brace back on as well as my socks and shoes. Each week I tell her how wonderful she is. "It's an hour of pure relaxation for me," she assures me. "And, besides, this way we get to see each other at least once a week. You put up with so much and I love doing it."

"I agree that I put up with a lot, especially today," I confessed. "I was going to tell you earlier when you were massaging my feet. All morning long, I worked on setting up my pills for the next two weeks. I kept knocking over the pill containers, had trouble picking up the pills and putting them back where they belong."

"Stop," Bridgit said. "Martha, I would be happy to do the pills for you. I know I can do it a lot easier and faster than you can. We'll start in two weeks. I'll allow time to set up the pills before we do your foot massage." What a friend. Bridgit now comes every week to massage my feet and every other week, comes earlier to do my pills. WOW!

As she leaves, I give Bridgit a hug and say, "Who says that Parkinson's is all bad. After all, if it weren't for Parkinson's, you wouldn't be massaging my feet the way you do."

"Martha," she says, looking me straight in the eye, "It's a very small contribution that I can make. You put up with a lot."

I agree.

St. Agnes Reunion

Happiness is not a matter of events, it depends
upon the tides of the mind.

— *Alice Meynell*

In my 2013 Christmas letter to one of my St. Agnes friends, I wrote: "Joyce, in your Christmas card you mentioned I was very sick. I don't feel sick at all. I am just very limited in what I can do and I fall a lot. My balance stinks. Other than that, I am fine. Parkinson's is the disease I have, but I prefer to think of it as a condition, albeit a not so fun condition where you slowly rot away. But I am still the same old Mopsy."

One of the highlights of 2013 was hosting my 51st high school reunion with Tessa, my roommate and best friend from St. Agnes School in Albany, New York. When I reached my old friend at her home in San Francisco and started to bounce my crazy idea off her, Tessa didn't hesitate. "Let's do it," she said simply.

Most of us chose not to attend the official 50th reunion because St. Agnes was no longer the school that we graduated from in 1962. It had been an Episcopal girl's school founded in 1870. It closed its doors just over a century later in 1975. Only the statue of St. Agnes with her lamb, which stood at the entryway of the school, had survived its demolition. Our alma mater had merged with Kenwood Academy, to become Doane Stuart School.

But St. Agnes was the place many of us had formed lifelong friendships, connections I needed now more than ever, connections I was determined to keep. So why not have a second 50th reunion here at my seaside home in Maine? To accomplish that, I knew I would need help and lots of it.

Soon after Christmas I started organizing the reunion for the very next fall with my former roomie's long-distance help. Tessa had set the precedent by hosting our 25th reunion when she had been living on the East Coast, a reunion well-attended. Meanwhile, another former classmate, Wynne Edwards, jumped in to help with the mailing list. Since I could no longer write legibly or type on my computer keys accurately, Wynne's help was essential. Whenever I needed to communicate with my classmates,

Wynne stepped in to let everyone know what was going on.

Getting organized took a lot of time and effort, more than I expected. I was concerned that I didn't have enough energy to pull it off. My balance in particular could cause serious problems. I was falling so much that I stopped counting. Looking forward, I had no idea what my physical state would be. But, I forged ahead.

Ideally, I wanted to find a place where everyone could stay together, but who was coming and how many? I had to pin down when people were arriving, how they were traveling, if they were carpooling. Would stairs be an issue? Were there bathrooms nearby? Did anyone have special dietary needs?

It was a big job. But as the year wore on, and my PD symptoms became more obvious, I found myself thinking more about the coming reunion and less about IT. I was buried with lists of things to do including the to-do list for me in Tessa's handwriting.

For the reunion we had the warm, sunny, blue sky days I had hoped for and the crowd I had longed for. Although staying under one roof was not an option, once again, my friends and neighbors came through, providing beds and places for dinner.

It started with a casual supper on Thursday with fourteen women gathering at my house sitting around talking. Most of us hadn't seen each other in 51 years.

Activities the next day included a picnic along the water and hike among the ruins of a local civil war fort, and dinner at my friend Marcia's house, which has gorgeous views of the harbor and where you can catch the sunset. Dinner was cooked by three classmates. We had a special guest, my mother who was from the class of 1933 at St. Agnes. She happened to live nearby. That evening she wore a crown of flowers made by Marcia.

Saturday we went on a boat trip around the harbor and then feasted on a lobster dinner. After lobster and corn, we went to A.M.'s house to enjoy the ocean before the sky turned dark. It was an evening under the stars, sitting around a fire pit sharing stories and singing familiar hymns that we'd learned at St. Agnes. Our favorite one was "For All the Saints."

On Sunday we met back at my house for breakfast and people left slowly because they hated to see the reunion end.

Reaching Out

"They are not gone who live in the hearts they left behind."

— *Unknown*

Folding chairs had been set up and crammed together in the upstairs room of the Kittery Art Association to accommodate as many people as possible. Just as the play reading was about to begin, a man about my age, his shoulders stooped and his head down, shuffled into the room. Spotting the last three seats in the crowded room, the man and his two friends sat down right in front of my friend Betty and me.

As the play reading began, I leaned over and whispered to her, "I think he has Parkinson's. What do you think?" Betty shrugged, her eyes focused on the play. "I'm going to ask him at the intermission," I whispered again, giving her a gentle poke to get her attention.

"You can't do that," she said, now turning to me with a frown. "What happens if he doesn't have it? You might embarrass him."

"I'll take my chances," I whispered once more, ignoring her look.

At intermission, I tapped this man on his shoulder, introduced myself, and asked, "Do you have Parkinson's? I think we may have something in common." A big smile crossed his face. We talked through the entire intermission. I had been living with a Parkinson's diagnosis for twenty-one years at the time.

His was a recent diagnosis, this new friend, David, told me, adding he knew nothing about the disease except that he didn't like it. "No, that's wrong," he said with a deep sigh, staring at me for a long moment, his eyes clouding with tears. "My diagnosis has been absolutely devastating," he muttered finally. He had been physically active his entire life, he said, a regular at the gym in the winter, kayaking every summer, loving basketball with his four grandchildren.

As the lights dimmed, announcing the end of the intermission, the man clasped my hand and said, "I've never even met anyone who has Parkinson's. You're the first. I'm so delighted to talk with you."

Gripping his hand in return, I promised to call him in a few weeks, and we quickly exchanged phone numbers. "We'll get together and talk some more," I said. "I promise."

As Betty was taking her seat, she heard the last part of our conversation. "I'm flabbergasted," she said, shaking her head once again. "You amaze me, Martha. You'll talk to anyone."

I nodded and smiled, saying nothing. What Betty would never know is that while we Parkinsonians need and desperately value friends like her to lean on, we need a special kind of support that only other Parkinsonians can provide.

Bluebirds

"Be happy for this moment. This moment is your life."
— *Omar Khayyam*

I opened one eye, then the other. I reached for my remote control to open the blinds while lying in bed. It was a sunny, ten-degree day. I preferred staying put in my warm bed, watching the song-birds come to my window feeder, the ball feeder, and the rhododendron bush.

The rhododendron sits in my yard near the deck, over-looking Chauncey Creek, my tidal treasure. My bush is huge and bears deep pink flowers each June. If you knew how songbirds and bluebirds talk, they would tell you my bush is their sanctuary. They are constantly flying in and out

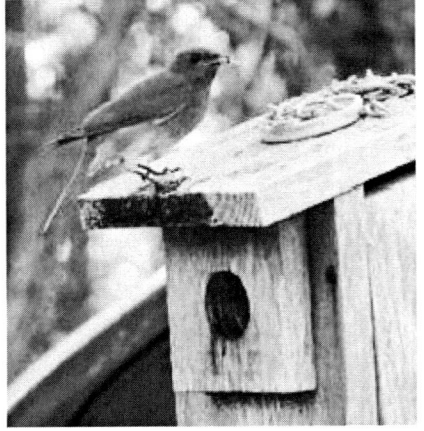

of it. They also love my pear tree with its craggy limbs and branches, looking like an old man bent over with arthritis— or maybe like me with my Parkinson's.

Suddenly I catch a glimpse of something. Can it be? I sit up as quickly as my stiff body will allow. Now, I sit on the edge of my bed and stare. The shape is right. It has an orange, puffed-out chest, and I see a touch of blue. It perches on a branch, sticking out from the rhododendron bush, and doesn't budge. It looks like it's frozen in place.

I must start moving and take my medicine or I will be frozen, too, but I can't take my eyes off this bird. Finally my patience is rewarded. This bird has left the branch and flown to the feeder where I can admire her soft, muted blue tones. I know the male in his iridescent blueness won't be far behind. You would think I had won the lottery.

I know one of my bluebird couples will return in a few weeks to check out my birdhouse. They have their own schedule. But I have seen them, and I must have patience, a characteristic I desperately need for dealing with Parkinson's.

I have to share my news. I called my friend Judy in Connecticut that very minute. "Judy," I squealed to my long-time camp friend, "I've just seen Jesus!" She knew exactly what I meant, and five days later, a box arrived from some outfit in Ohio with the words "Keep Refrigerated" emblazoned in big, bold letters on the sides. I tore open the package. Inside were five thousand meal worms, alive and squirming all over each other.

I called her again. "Judy, I'm not sure whether I should say, 'thank you' or not," I said with a laugh. "Who counts them anyway? And do you truly tuck these worms in with your food in your fridge?"

"Anything for bluebirds, she said. "Bluebirds love 'em."

Watching my birds has become an endless new source of entertainment for me. Because I can no longer drive, I don't get out as I did before. Money I used to spend on going out, eating out, going to the Music Hall or the movies now goes to the birds. I feel sad when I am not included when my friends and others go out on the town, but I know my limitations. Now, I turn to my birds.

Word is out that we have the best birdseed money can buy and it's always in good supply. I just wish my blue-birds would return. I'm trying to be patient.

Women's Walk/Bummed Out

"I tell you, in this world being a little crazy
helps to keep you sane."

— *Zsa Zsa Gabor*

Duy the 2016 presidential elections, my friends and I learned that political rallies are not designed for people with physical challenges. Yes, I was entering my twenty-fifth year surviving Parkinson's, but YES, I wanted to continue living my life. Bernie Sanders, Hillary Clinton and Maggie Hassan, the Governor of New Hampshire, were being highlighted at a rally in nearby Portsmouth where Bernie planned to announce his support for Hillary Clinton for president.

We got there, but it was disastrous for us both. It was a wicked hot day. A.M. and I learned the hard way that attending rallies was not good for people like me.

A.M. dropped me at the front door of the local high school where the rally was being held. Before she drove off to park, she made sure I had help from one of the volunteers, and we agreed to find each other when the rally ended.

Having Parkinson's won me a seat in the front row, but there were so many people there, many standing in front of me, that I couldn't see Bernie, Hillary or Maggie. Nor could I stand up because there was nothing to hold on to. I was a captive there. I kept looking behind me for A.M. who I thought would be easy to spot with her gorgeous white hair. No way. When she finally parked her car and got to the rally, having walked back almost a mile in the heat, she was directed to the opposite side of the gym, and we never found each other. Our cell phones didn't work, but luckily, Chuck and Lynn Hatch, a couple from church, drove me home.

So there I was six months later, on January 21st, 2017, Inauguration Day. Millions of us were determined to express our outrage at the results of the election in November. "The March for Women."

My heart was wanting to be a part of everything, but my body was screaming, "NO." I wasn't used to sitting on the sidelines. No one called that day to say, "Hey, Martha, let's go to the Women's March in Portsmouth." I felt alone and lonely. I had a pity party all by myself, something I rarely do. It wasn't until noontime I realized I could watch the march on TV, improving my spirits exponentially.

Over time, as I've become increasingly debilitated, I've also become high maintenance. My friends are willing and able to get my walker in and out of their cars, but I know it's a pain for them. They get me to my appointments, my writing group and my church. But these days, I would never want—or expect—anyone to take me to a gathering as large as that Women's March, which was expected to be huge. I recognized after my fiasco with A.M. that I could no longer participate in large events. And it was a bummer.

Now, before even thinking about attending these size-able occasions, I must ask: How many people will be there? Will there be seating? Is there a chance of violence? How will I do being jostled?

Two days later, as my neurologist was going through his regular checklist, he looked up and asked, "Are you depressed at all?"

"I was on Saturday," I said, trying to sound lighthearted. "I wanted to go to the Women's March in Portsmouth. I try never to let Parkinson's get in my way, but on Saturday, it did big time."

Dr. Kleinman rolled his chair right up to me and said with a smile, "You weren't remotely the only one who was depressed on Saturday."

The Final Indignity

"The trick in life is learning how to deal with it."
— Helen Mirren

I was overwhelmed by all the people I didn't know who came to my house—all on the same day. Well, it wasn't exactly like that, but it felt like that.

In this, my twenty-eighth year of Parkinson's, my life has been turned upside down, and I feel as though my life in my wonderful seaside town will never be the same again.

Suddenly new names are emblazoned on the weekly schedule that is emailed to me every Friday by Extended Family, a local agency that provides home care for people like me.

Wait a minute here. I can't have all these people suddenly become a part of my life, just to keep me safe. It's too much. Those of us with Parkinson's don't need additional stress fired at us.

———— // ————

It all began with what I called a "family intervention" with my daughter Katie, my son Stephen on speaker phone, brother Steve, and Mary, the clinical nurse from Extended Family. This was a serious meeting.

The focus was entirely on me—my falling and the rapid decline in my health. So much love and caring. But what did they want? For me to go to assisted living? Leave my Kittery home where I watch the birds every day? Where I have found so much peace and happiness?

Not necessarily, but they were desperate for me to acknowledge that I needed more help. Every year for the past fifteen, I had participated in the Parkinson's Unity Walk and could walk two miles. I couldn't do that today.

Still, it has taken a lot of adjustment to get used to what I agreed to at the family meeting. Round-the-clock care, 24/7. Yes, it's okay to have a stranger help me get dressed in the morning or get to bed. But how would you feel if you had a complete stranger standing next to you when you took a shower? And how would you feel to have someone always around, after many years of staunch independence?

But with the 24/7 care, I get to still have my ocean, the garden, and those birds and the peace and quiet of my Kittery home. Yes, sometimes the waves tumble around me, but I have to admit it is better to be upright as I watch them.

ONE YEAR LATER

July 26, 2020

The first six months were tough. I was used to having my generous friends and part-time caregivers help me out, but the intervention made me realize I was worse off than I thought I was.

I needed to expand my care from part-time to full time with Extended Family. At the beginning of these changes, many people were coming and going. I felt like I was training them.

When we managed to find the right fit, I came to appreciate those who have greatly helped me: Connie, Maria and Jen. I finally have adjusted to having professional help from Extended Family. I've come to accept that I truly need round-the-clock care. I couldn't manage by myself.

I have been using a walker or a wheelchair for a few years where I used to walk and run freely. Without help I can easily fall to the ground, and I could no longer get up or walk by myself. Then along came Jerry Parrota, home care physical therapist from York Hospital, who challenged me to walk again. He was magical and inspired me to exercise and walk every day. Now instead of being limited to just walking on the deck, I can walk up the driveway and down the road along the creek for a half- mile round trip.

I realize I need to keep that up. It's not realistic to think I can improve my symptoms without great effort. I need to keep the effort up in order to continue to walk, but Jerry provided hope and inspiration.

Epilogue

"When the unthinkable happens, the lighthouse is hope. Once we choose hope, everything is possible."
— Christopher Reeve

I have ended up where I was in childhood. My friends and caregivers help me tie my shoes, zipper my jacket. They get too frustrated watching me. Being able to laugh about it with them makes it possible.

These have been difficult times with the COVID-19 virus, making my life more isolated in many ways. However, it has reminded me that I guess you can say that I am lucky in one respect—one of Parkinson's few attributes is that is does not compromise one's immune system.

I never intended to write a book. Rather, it evolved from writing vignettes while participating in my writers' group. The vignettes were based solely on memories of events and circumstances and were grouped together in some semblance of order for this book. Most books with personal accounts of Parkinson's discuss at least some aspects of the science of the disease. I have chosen instead to share the everyday, the nuts and bolts of adjusting to the realities of Parkinson's in my daily life.

When I appreciate what I have, I rejoice for my family, my three "perfect" grandchildren, for my dear friends who include me in their activities, the church community that has given me so much and my beautiful home on the seacoast.

We're closing in on three decades since Parkinson's showed up. Although I'm now pretty much wheelchair bound and require twenty-four hour care, I have discovered a life well worth living.

Much of my determination and stamina come from lessons I learned at that girls' camp on Squam Lake in the White Mountains of New Hampshire. I became a camper there as an eleven-year-old and returned every year until I was old enough to become a councillor. Among those lessons learned was the value of nourishing long-term relationships.

My symptoms continue to develop as does my determination to record and share my experiences with millions of my fellow Parkinsonians who are faced with similar chal-lenges. I hope my writings have helped you.

Parkinson's has closed many doors, but it has opened at least as many. Take *that*, Parkinson's – and take *THAT*!

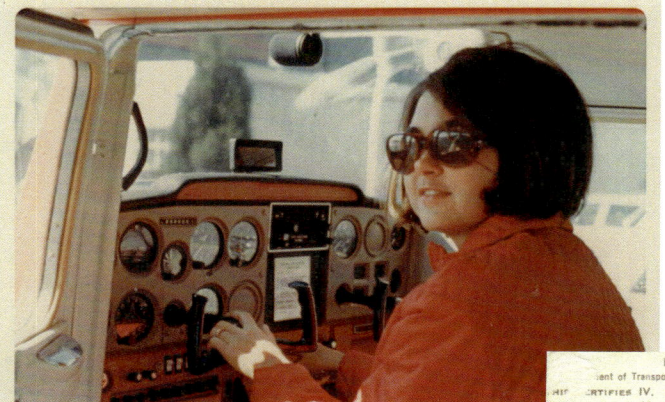

Back in the day...

At the controls.

I. UNITED STATES OF AMERICA

ent of Transportation- FEDERAL AVIATION ADMINISTRATION

CERTIFIES IV. MARTHA KOWAL CRAWFORD
THAT V. 70& HOPETON RD.
WILMINGTON DELAWARE 19807

| DATE OF BIRTH | HEIGHT | WEIGHT | HAIR | EYES | SEX | NATIONALITY |
| 05-11-44 | 64 IN. | 125 | BROWN | BLUE | F | USA |

IX. HAS BEEN FOUND TO BE PROPERLY QUALIFIED TO EXERCISE THE PRIVILEGES OF

II. PRIVATE PILOT III. CERT. NO. 2170255

RATINGS AND LIMITATIONS

XII. AIRPLANE SINGLE-ENGINE LAND#

XIII.

VII. *Martha K Crawford* X.
SIGNATURE OF HOLDER ADMINISTRATOR

X. DATE OF ISSUE: 06-03-72 VIII.

AC FORM 8060-2 (8-71)

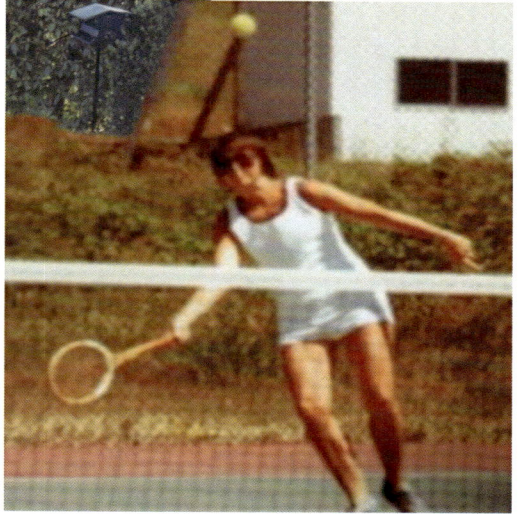

Poor form on this shot.

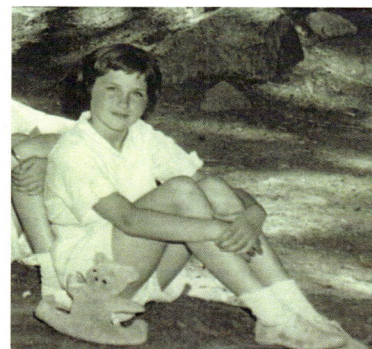

My first year at camp, age 11.

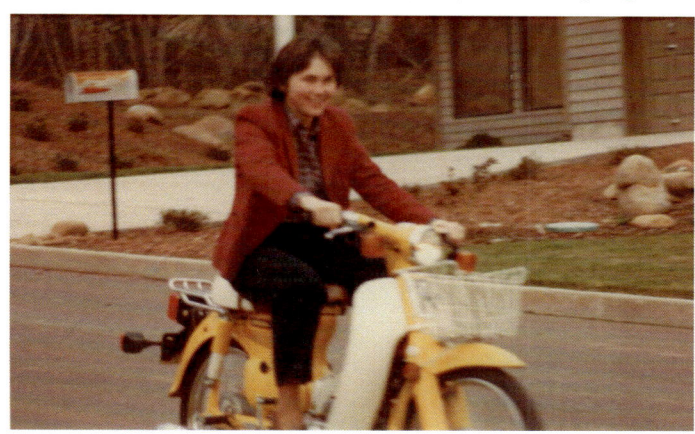

*Taking a ride on some-
body's motorbike.
Wowwee!*

Four generations...

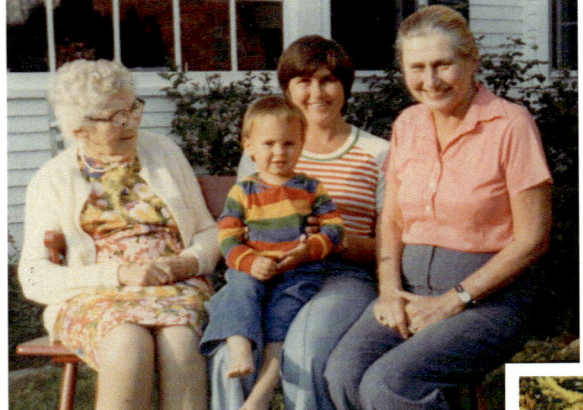

Four generations, c. 1978: my grandmother, Margret Carlisle Averill; Katharine Averill Crawford – Katie; Martha Ames Kowal Crawford – me; and my mother, Elizabeth Averill Kowal.

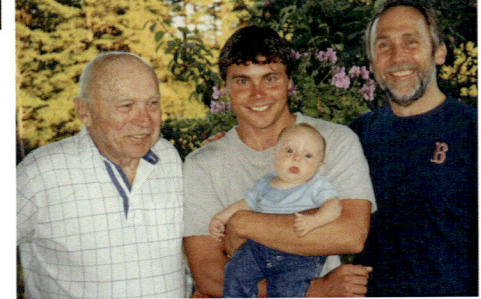

Four generations: my father, brother Steve, his son Kris and grandson Samual.

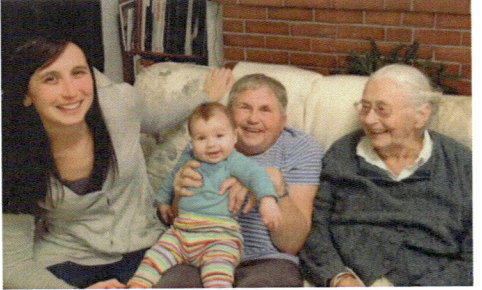

And another four generations: Katie, my granddaughter Anna in my arms, me and my mother.

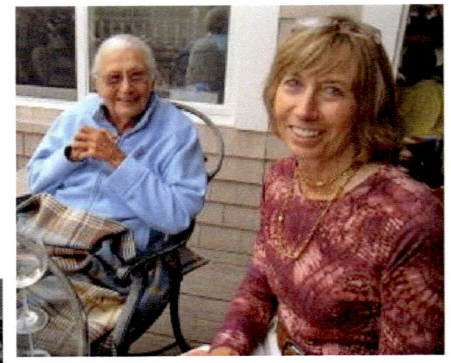

Mom and sister Susan.

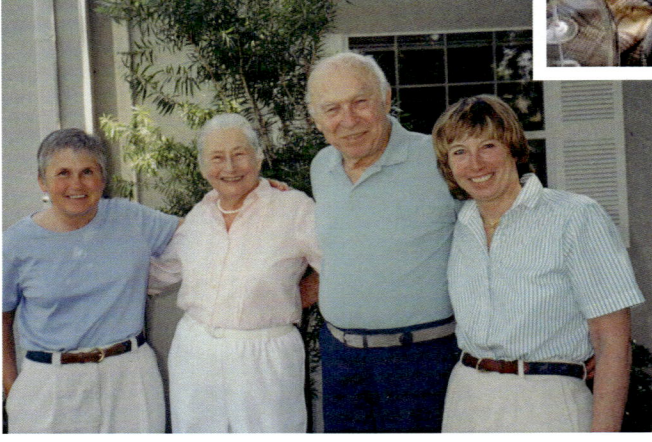

Me, Mom, Dad and sister Susan.

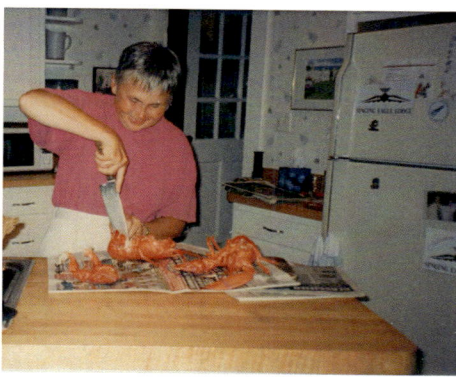

What people do in Maine – prepare lobster, cook lobster, consume lobster.

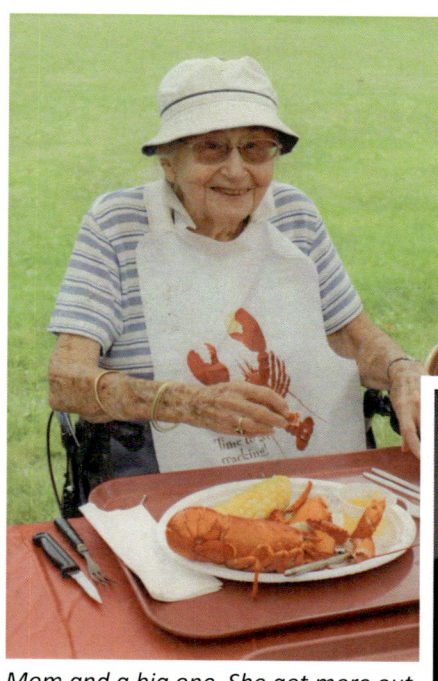

Mom and a big one. She got more out of a lobster than anyone I know.

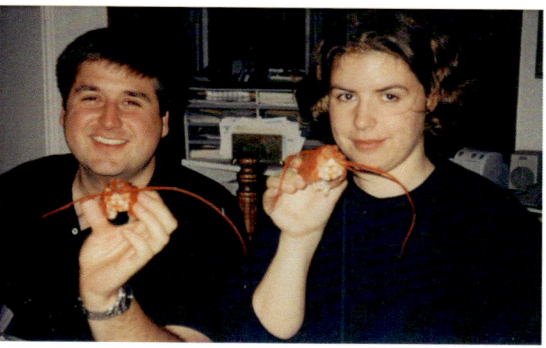

Stephen, Arabella and their lobsters.

Susan, Steve and me, and the Nubble Light, Cape Neddick, Maine.

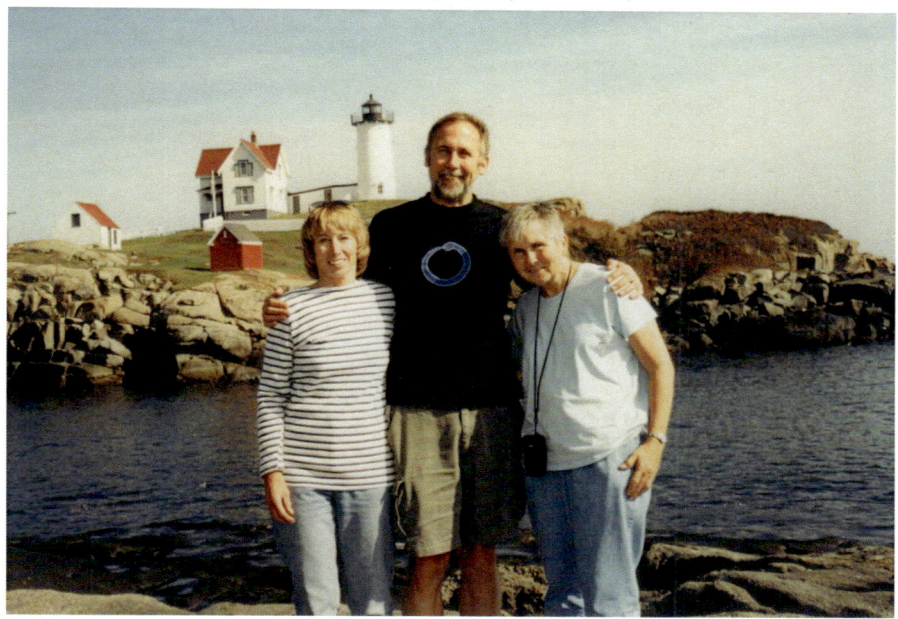

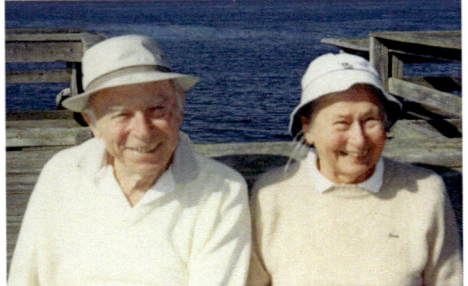

Dad and Mom enjoy the water.

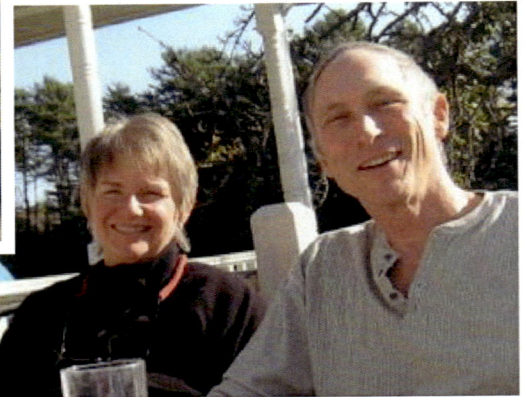

Brother Bob and his wife Pat.

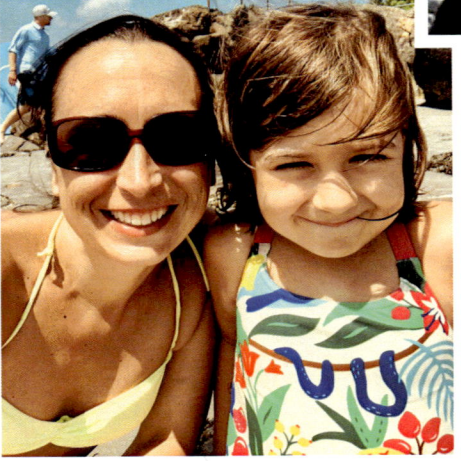

Daughter Katie and granddaughter Anna.

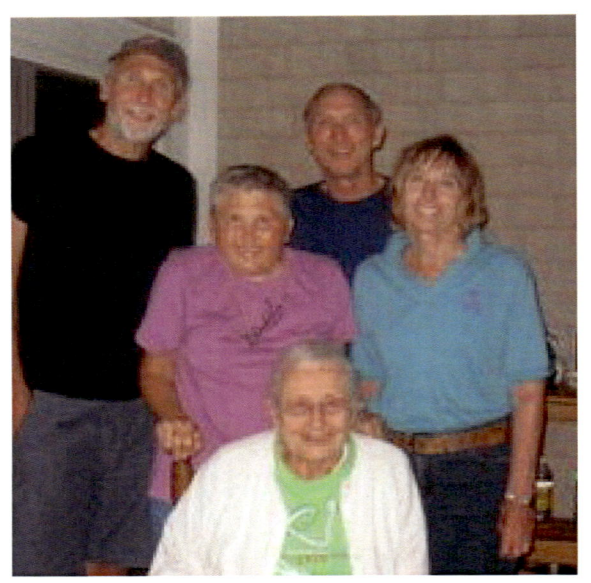

Dad and Mom on his 90th.

Steve, me, Bob, Susan and Mom.

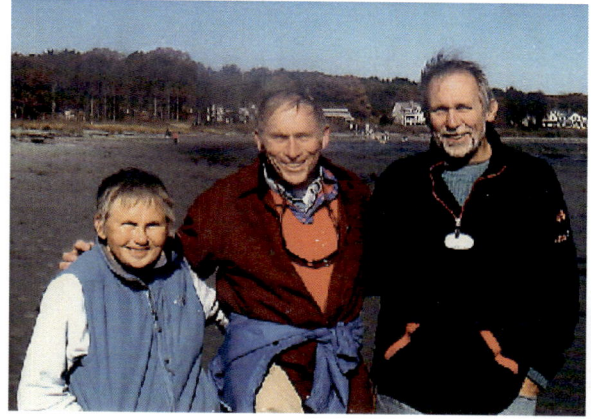

At at Sea Point Beach with my brothers Bob and Steve.

Alex giving Farmer Steve a hand.

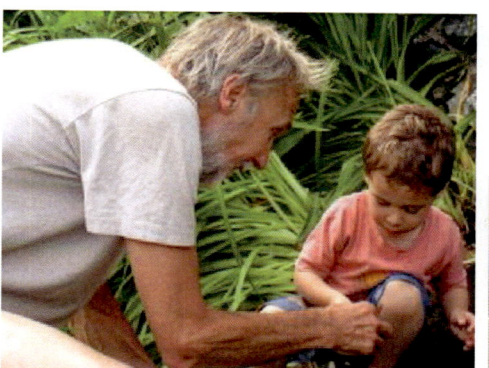

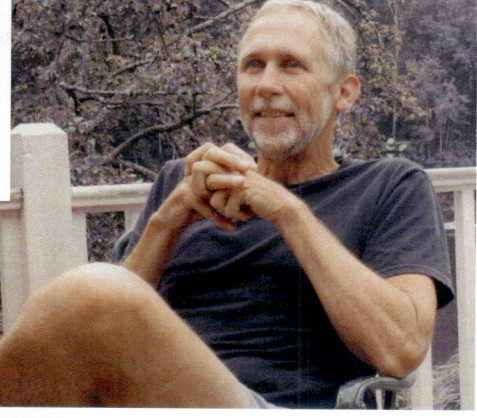

Steve hard at work.

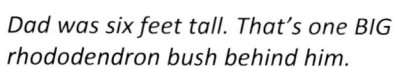

Steve relaxing.

Dad was six feet tall. That's one BIG rhododendron bush behind him.

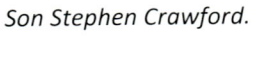
Son Stephen Crawford.

Stephen, Alex and Luke.

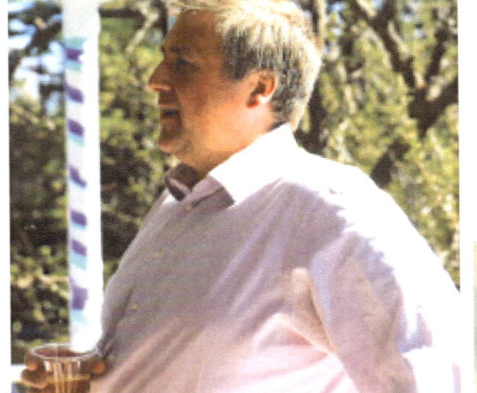

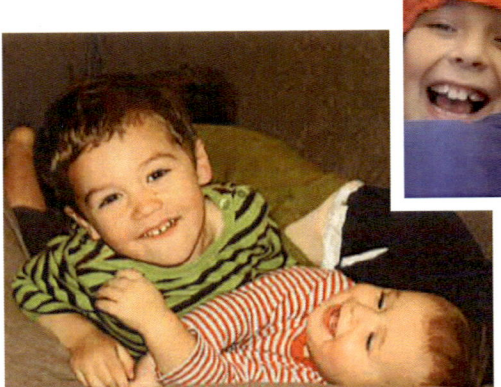

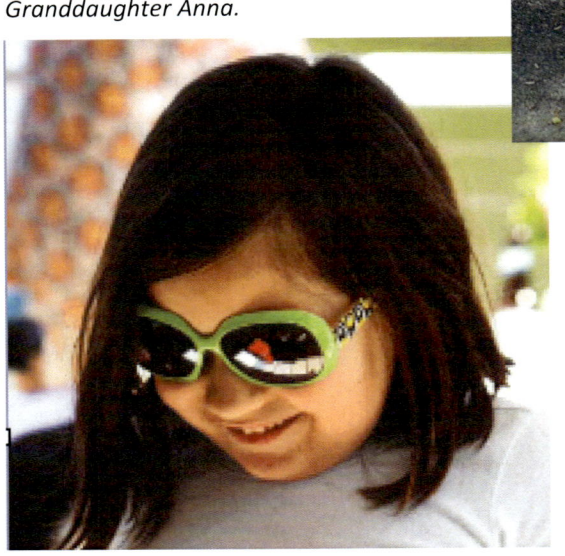

Grandsons Alex and Luke.

Granddaughter Anna.

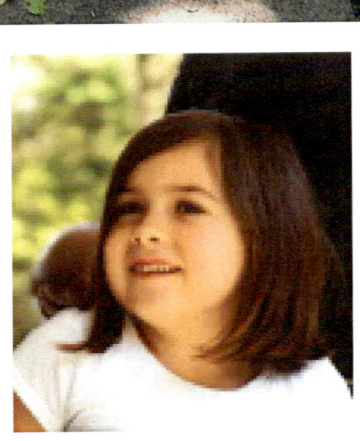

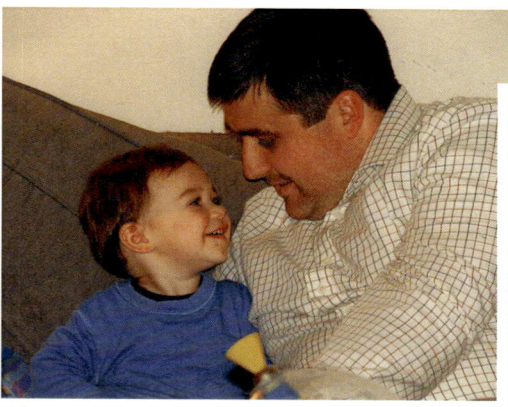

Alex and his dad.

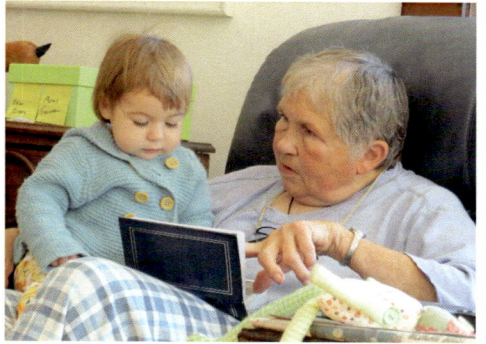

Anna and her Gami looking at pictures of animals from Africa.

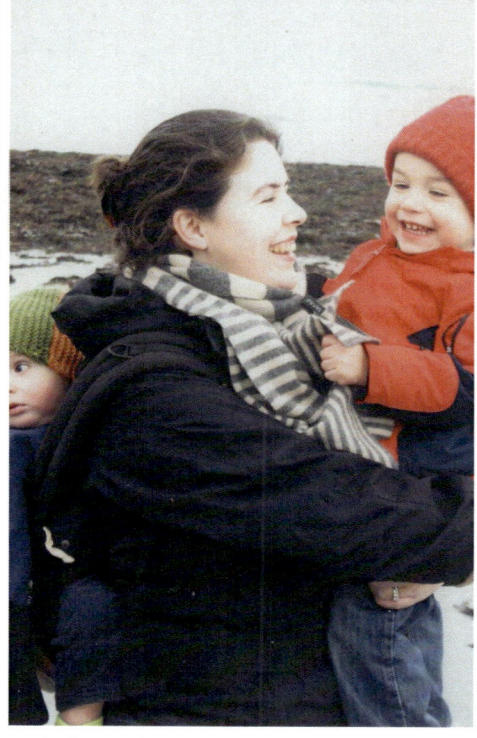

Arabella, with Alex in front and Luke tagging along on her back.

Daughter Katie and me, different occasions five years apart, same shirt.

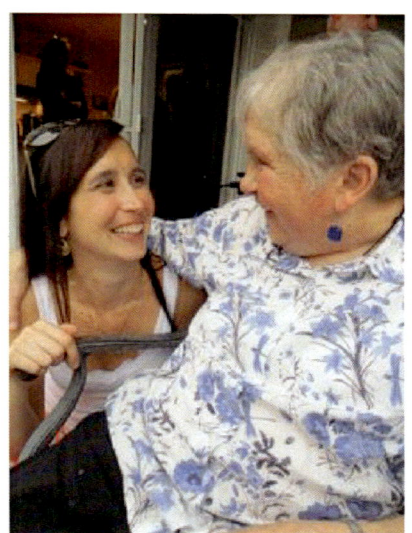

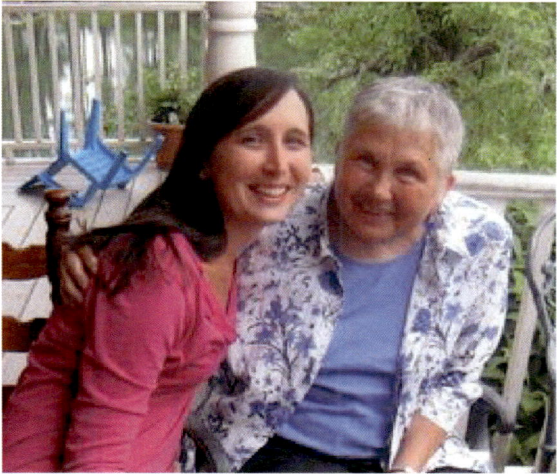

The annual Parkinson's Unity Walk in New York's Central Park

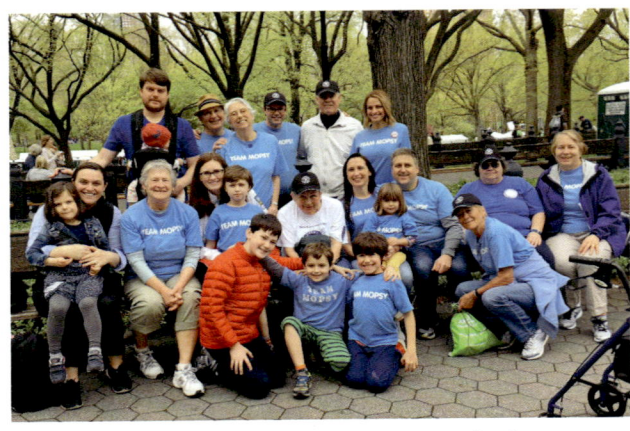

Team Mopsy, Alex and Luke in the front row.

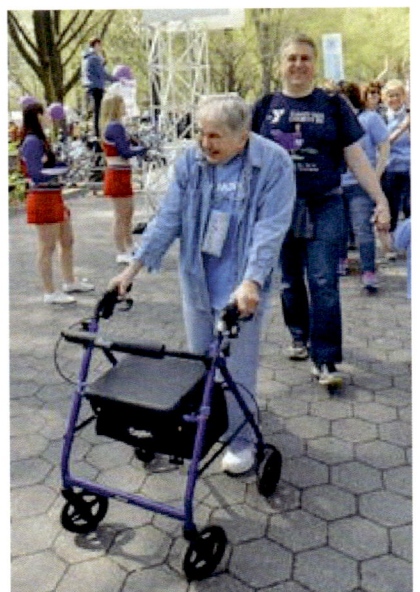

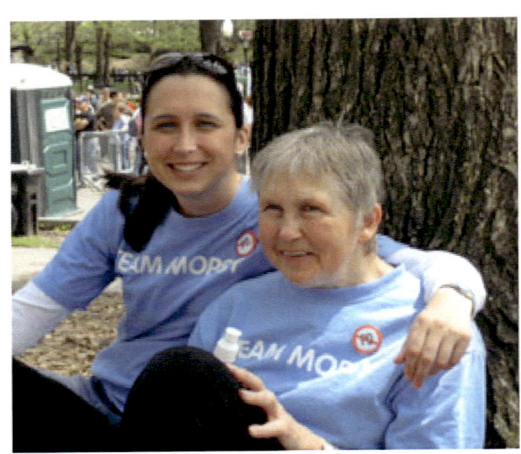

The second or third year, with Katie.

Stephen's got my back, encouraging me as we go.

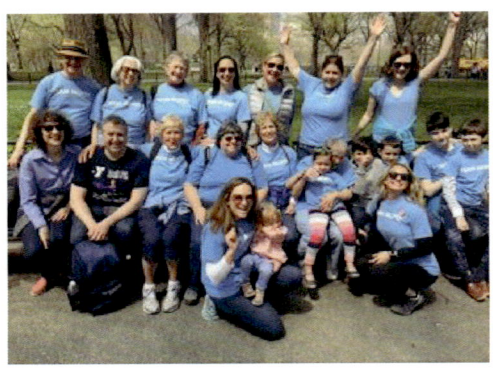

The whole team, 2011.

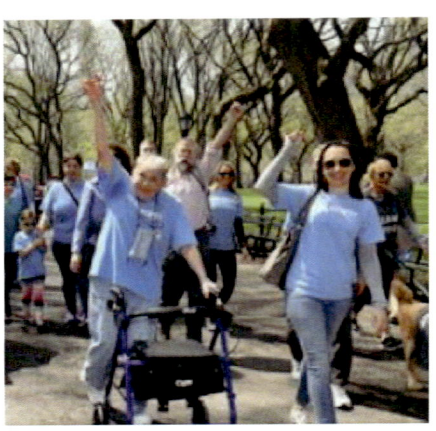

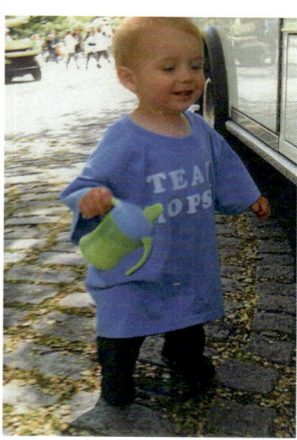

Luke, not quite two. It'll take him a couple of years to grow into that shirt.

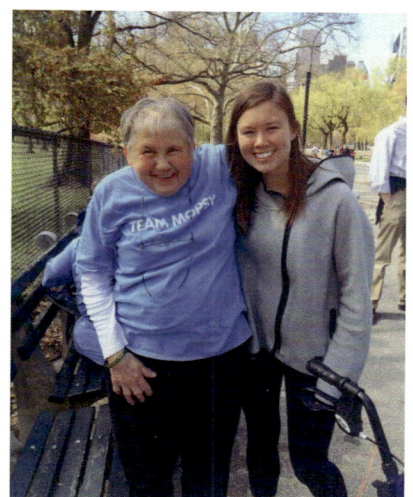

Emma, my first caretaker and a true friend. She quickly got me over my initial negativity of having a caretaker living in my house 24/7.

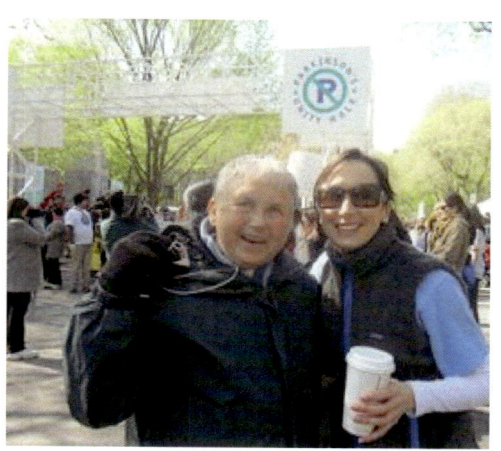

Katie and me celebrating yet again.

A Kittery Parkinson's Unity Walk.

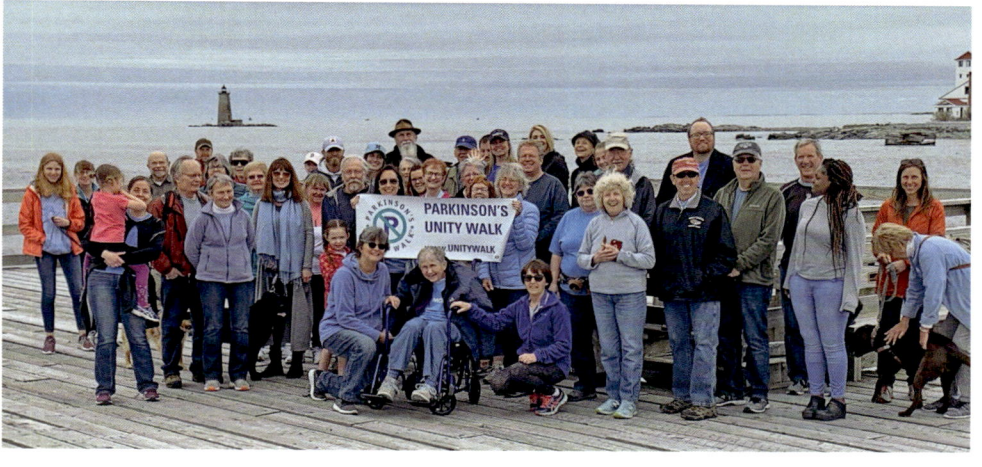

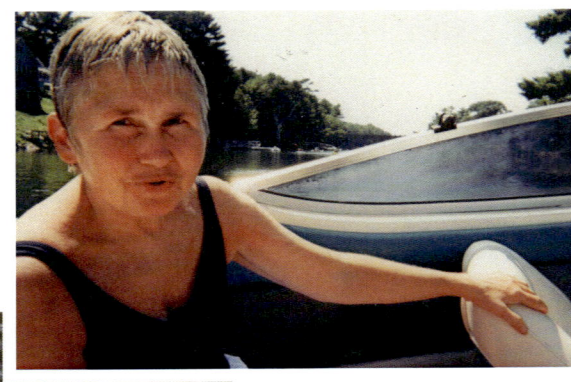

Relaxing on the creek.

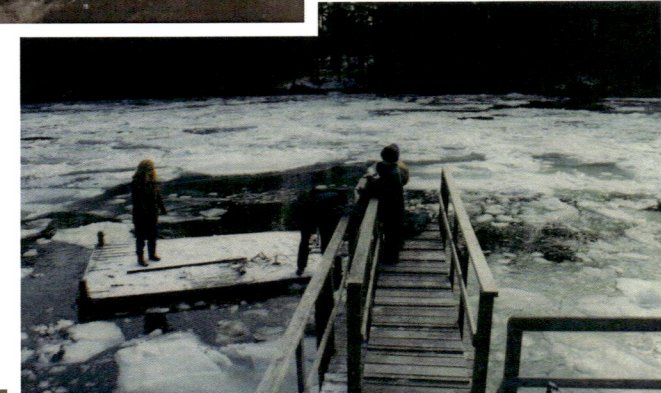

Enjoying swimming on the creek with Stephen.

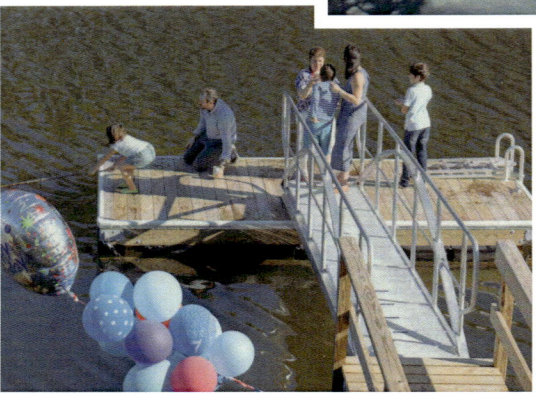

The creek come winter.

The view out the window on a spring or summer birthday.

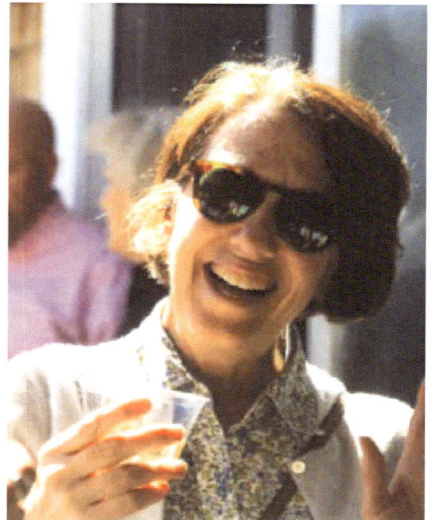

Marcye Philbrook, whose vignette begins on page 57.

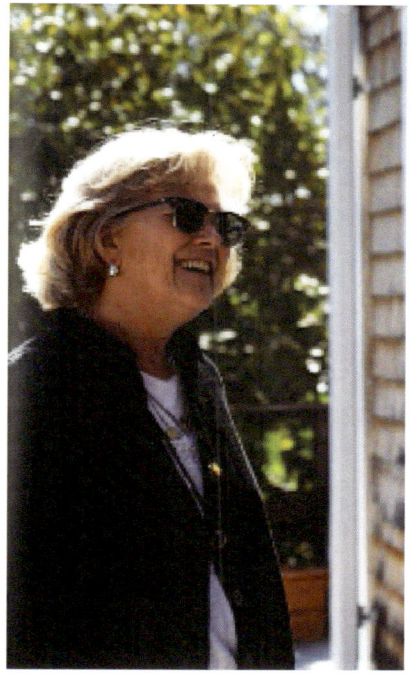

Linda Browning, my mortgage broker and friend.

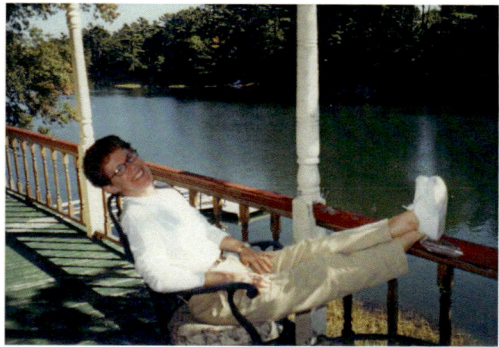

Ellie Gibeau, at her favorite spot on the deck.

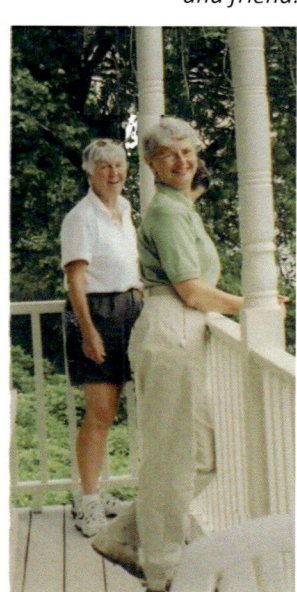

Two friends, A.M. McCurdy and Sara Rhoades.

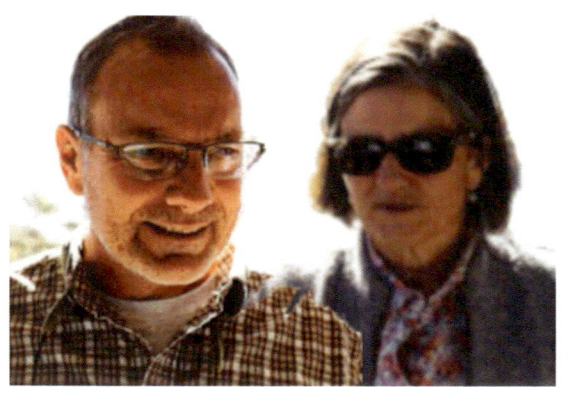

Sarah and Peter Drummond. Sarah is Marcia Gibbon's daughter.

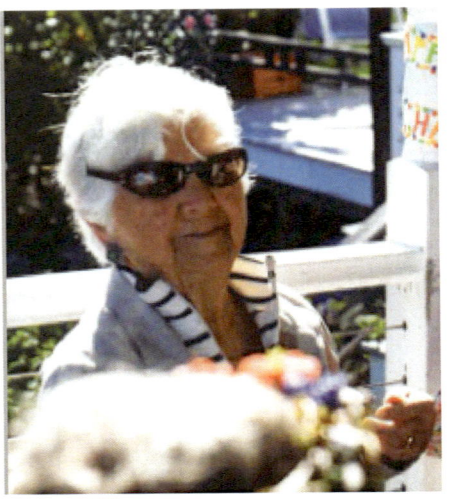

A.M. McCurdy, a wonderful presence.

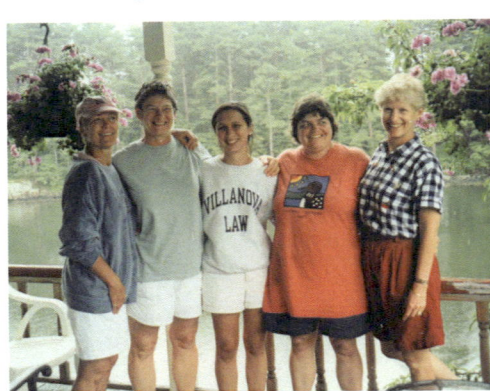

Kathe Chipman, my best friend growing up and my tennis cohort.

Lynn Luzzi and yours truly.

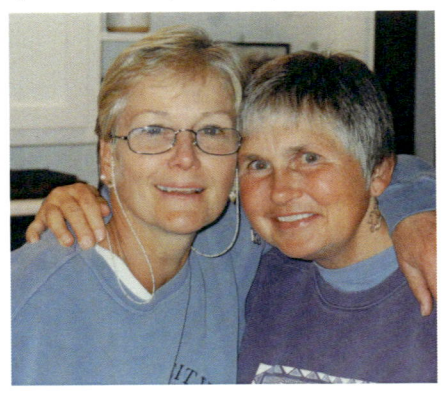

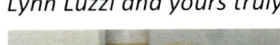

Camp friends Lynn Luzzi, Linda Briggs, Katie Crawford, Laura Livingston and Judy Hunter.

With Tessa Melvin. She has always been a kick to be around, a spark in my life.

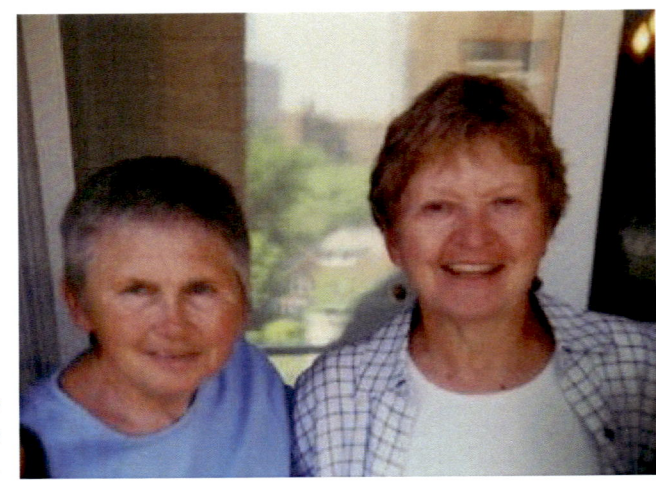

Liz Korabek-Emerson, helping me with the manuscript for this book.

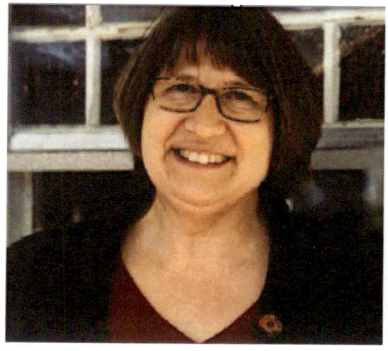

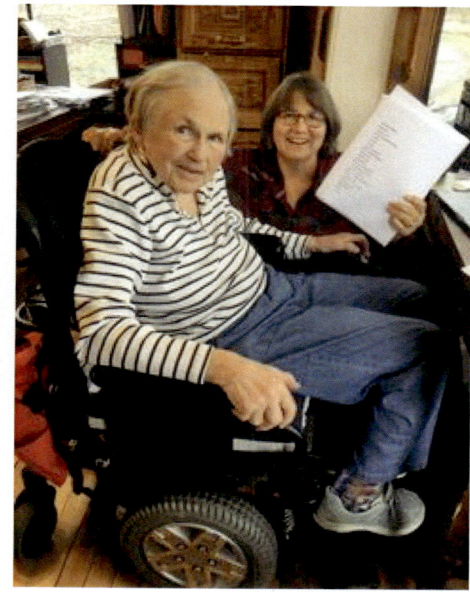

Sally Hirschberg, A.M. and her daughter Morgan McCurdy.

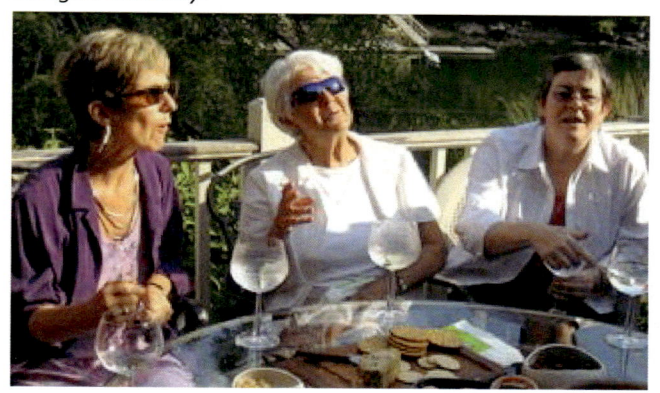

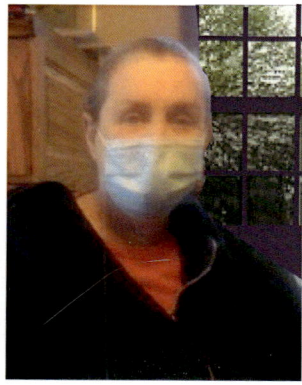

Nancy Grossman, editing in a mask.

Just two examples of wonderful times with A.M.

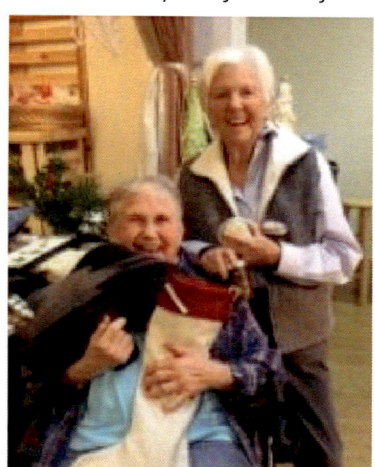

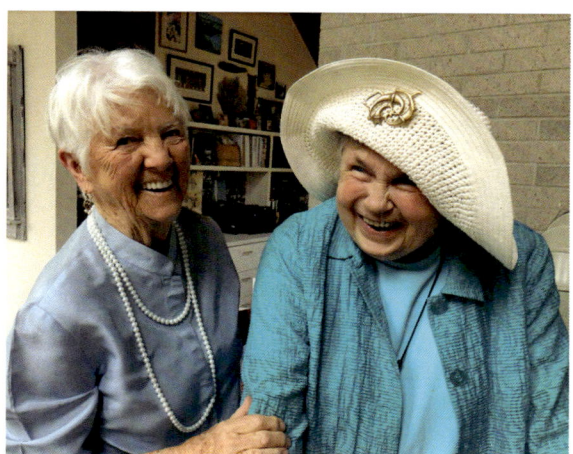

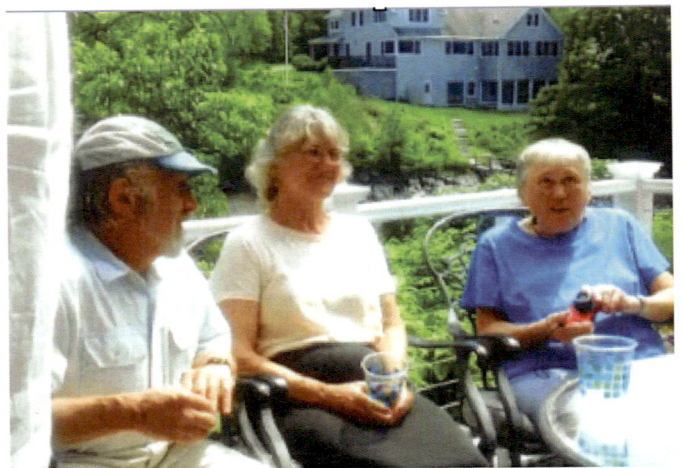

Rich and Bridgit Holzer live four houses down, caring neighbors.

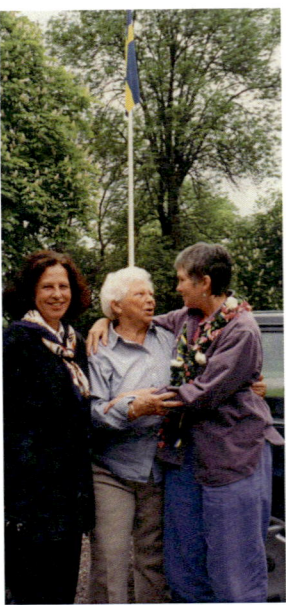

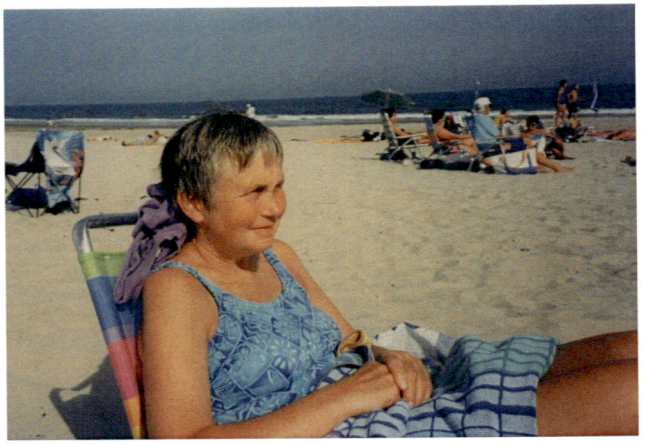

My Swedith "family." Lena Helgstrand and Annie Lindh, in Enköping, Sweden. This was just days after buying my Kittery home. I'd already planned the trip before my unplanned purchase.

Tessa Melvin and Bennett Swingle.

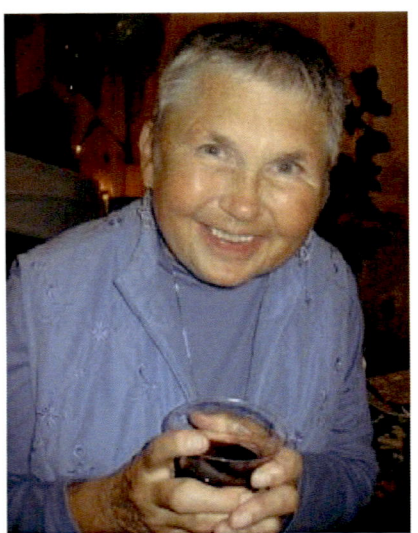

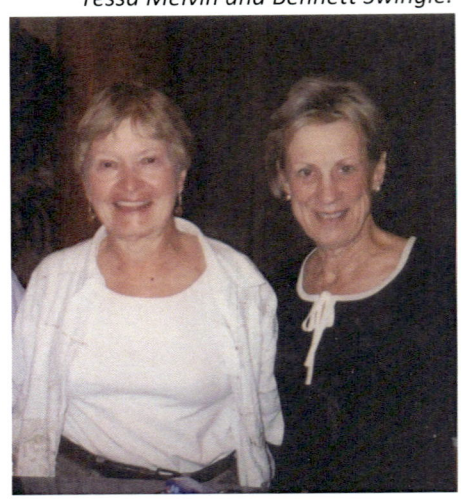

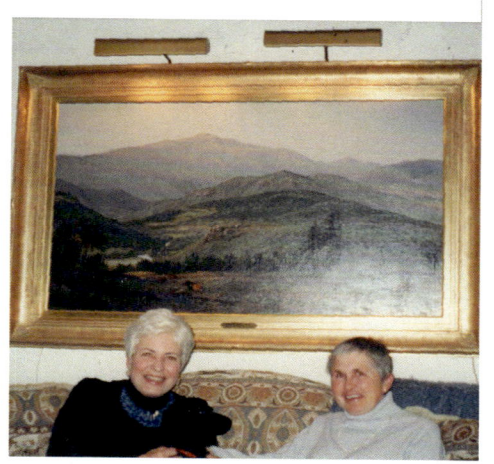

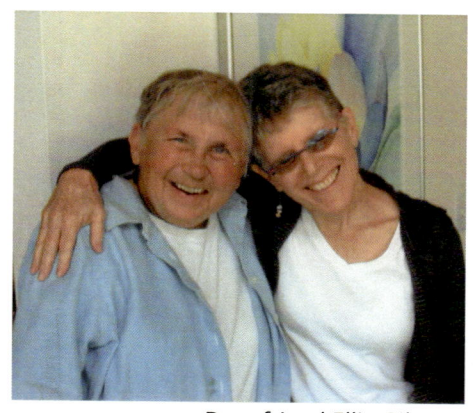

Dear friend Ellie Gibeau.

Marcia Vose, a family friend.

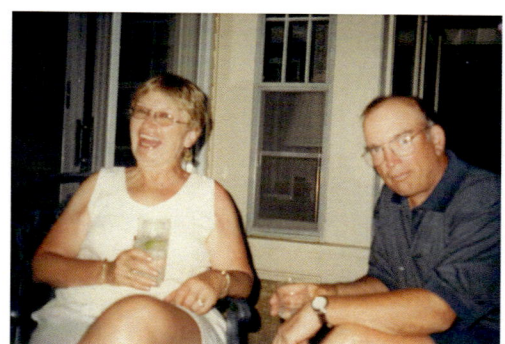

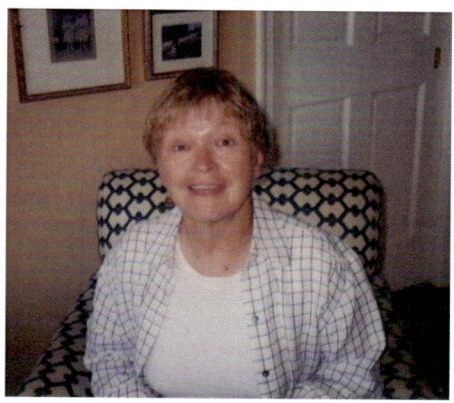

Tessa and her husband John, and Tessa herself.

With Bonnie Frisbee and Marcia Gibbons.   *Sally Donavon Goodrich in Afghanistan.*

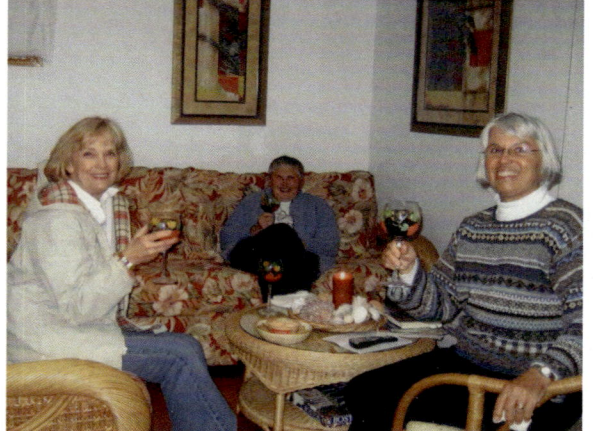

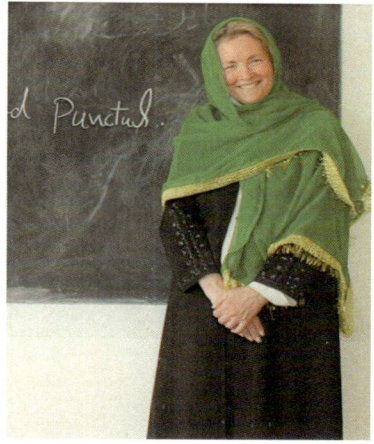

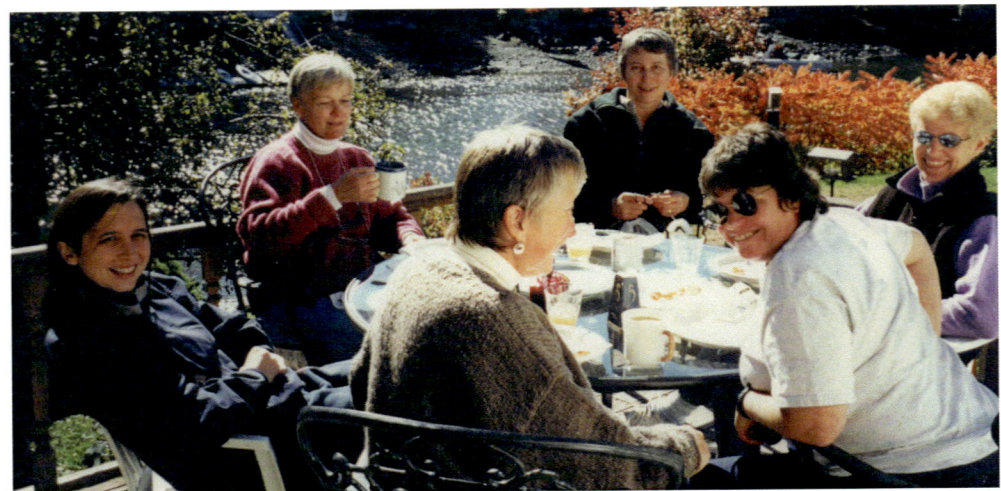

Clockwise from Katie on the left, and my camping family, Lynn Luzzi, Susan Kemp, Judy Hunter, Laura Livingston and me.

Judy Hunter, me and Lynn Luzzi.

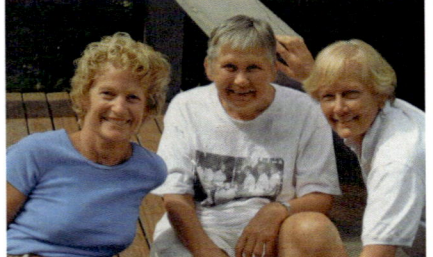

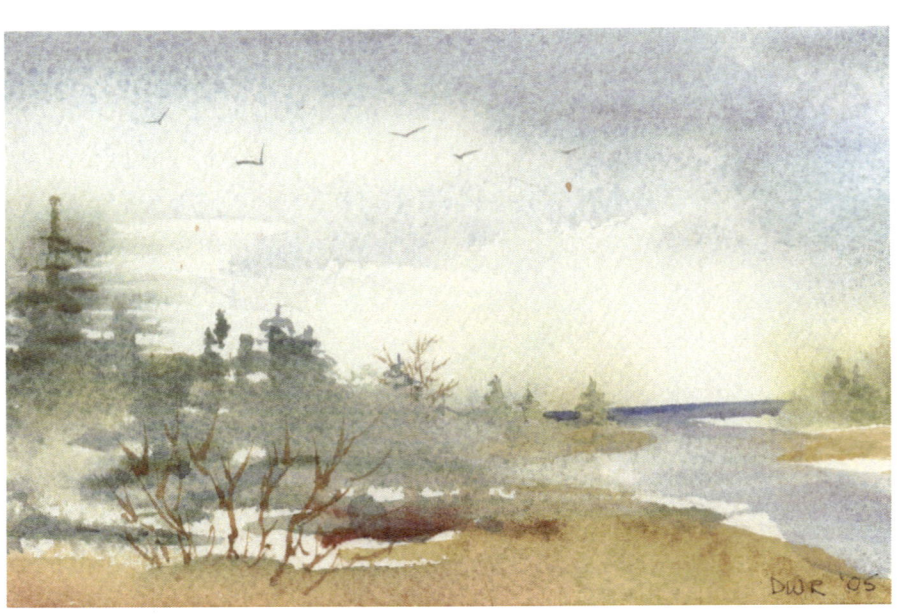

Laura Livingston, Judy Hunter and Peach Parke, bedded down on the floor for a sleepover.

Chauncey Creek painted from my deck by Kittery artist Debby Ronnquist.

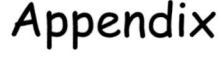

Appendix

Dad's Memorial Service

Henry J. Kowal

May 10, 1911—September 7, 2002

Well, Dad, no celebration of your life would be complete without mentioning your golf game.

First the statistics. While at Colgate in the early 1930s, you were named to the All-America Golf Team. You qualified for the National Amateur five times, won the Indiana State Championship twice, and won regional, city, and club championships too numerous to mention. In your prime, you held ten course records in New York State. And, beyond your prime, you twice won the New York Senior's Championship. And, remarkably, at the age of sixty-nine, you shot your age.

Steve and Bob, however, remember one time when you were too good. They recall attending an awards ceremony after the club championship one year. After eyeing the awards on display, with great disappointment, they asked, "Couldn't you have come in second this time?" The winner's award was yet another silver tray. The runner's up award was a new television set!

Dad, your life was like your golf game—top notch. You were a natural. As a scratch golfer, you shot straight down the fairway, chipped with great finesse, and had an incredible touch with putting. As good as you were, though, you always said golf was just a game. But through golf you taught us about life. You were a weekend golfer who never practiced, only played. That taught us to live life for real, not just practice it. You, thankfully, lived a full, healthy, and meaningful life to the ripe old age of ninety-one.

You gave us other messages too.

- Keep your eye on the ball. Don't look up. Message: Stay focused on whatever you're doing.

- Swing easy and let the club head do the work. You taught us about trust.

- Follow through. Follow through in life as well as on the course.

- Then there was one piece of advice that Steve remembers, but I don't. Be sure to wash your balls every once in a while.

I remember with great fondness as a kid going in summer evenings with you to hit some golf balls or to play a few holes. It was always a special time even though your coaching wasn't always very subtle. In exasperation, you'd exclaim, "You've got all that short grass in front of you, yet you insist on hitting into the long grass, on either side." Life's lesson learned was shoot straight, stay in the short grass, and you'll stay out of trouble. But the four of us did occasionally have some rough spots in our lives and, without reservation, you were always there to encourage and support us, and help us move back to the short grass.

Although you consistently drilled the ball straight down the fairway, you always said your short game, chipping and putting, was as important as your long game. Through that, you taught us that the small things in life often mattered more than the big showy things.

You were always modest about your accomplishments. You also were never too full of importance, as shown by the time you caddied for our cousin, Peter Hill, at the New York State junior boys qualifying tournament. You, needless to say, made an indelible impression on Peter, who was around age 12 at the time.

I remember my first birdie, probably my only birdie— it was a robin. We walked to the robin and you gave me your sweater in which to wrap it. We picked up our clubs and drove home. The robin didn't make it, but my remembrance of your sensitivity did and it still lives with me today.

At Carlmont during the summer, you would hit golf balls into the Ogunquit River at high tide and then we would go down at low tide and pick up the balls for you. You made it fun and we took great delight in counting the balls we found. I think you had a little bit of Tom Sawyer in you.

One summer, when you came up to Moody for a week or so, you learned of a golf tournament in Portland and entered it. The problem was you had neither golf clubs nor golf shoes with you. But, that didn't stop you. You borrowed some clubs and simply wore your white Ked sneakers. You came close to winning the tournament and were a sensation on the front page of the Portland sports section. Featured was a photo of you on the green wearing your white Ked sneakers! With that, you taught us that substance is more important that pretense, that you should be your own person and not worry about what others think. You also taught us to appreciate what you have and do the best you can with what you have. You, together with Mom, truly taught us the way we should live our lives.

As much as you loved golf, what you loved the most was Mom, the four of us, your grandchildren, and your one great grandchild. We cherish you for the love you continually gave us, and we loved you more than you can ever know.

Well, Dad, you've played your last eighteen, and you've moved on to a different round, gone to a different course. Just know we're putting along behind you and miss you greatly. We'll keep our eye on the ball for you.

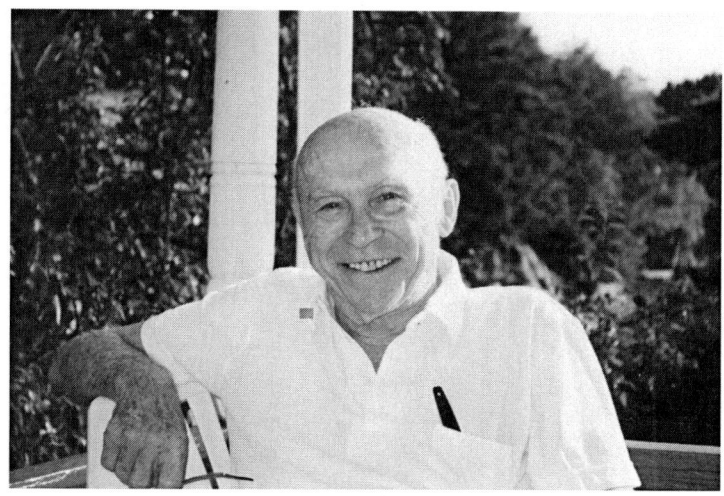

A Musing on Cookie Dough

Sent to my young friend, Hannah, for whom I served as a mentor in our church community.
— Easter Sunday 2008

"Faith is the force of life." — Tolstoy
"So is cookie dough." — Martha

Together we've made cookie dough, we've eaten cookie dough and with what was left, we've made some cookies along the way. We baked them as we discussed life.

Faith is like cookie dough, a mix of good things. The ingredients by themselves, however, aren't too tasty. Who would want to eat a spoonful of flour, or salt? Yuk! Our faith, at times, is like that. We struggle with bits and pieces of it. And, we don't get there easily. Sometimes the ingredients just aren't quite right. Just as we test and try new recipes, we test our beliefs in God and about God. Our faith grows as we face challenges, ask questions, doubt, learn, and reflect. As we throw ingredients into the bowl and that wonderful mix of cookie dough comes together, so does the strength of our beliefs.

We're blessed to have a church community like ours. Again, just as cookie dough is a mix of many ingredients, we come together as a mix of people of all ages, different backgrounds, and a variety of beliefs in God. Being connected to the church, like a recipe, gives us a framework to live by and the courage to question. We enjoy and feel love and support as we grow in faith and as we seek our very own path in life.

Hannah, may you experience fully the many paths that open to you. Keep making those cookies. And, I need not tell you, take big bites of cookie dough along the way.

My Happy Place

By Ellie Gibeau

My "happy place" is a hundred-year-old New Englander perched on Chauncey Creek in Kittery Point, Maine. It's where I go in my mind when I'm having a bad day. It's also where I spend many of my summer (and fall) vacations.

The property belongs to my friend Martha who bought it in 1998, just before I moved to Sarasota. Immediately after she closed with the bank, she left on a trip to Sweden. While she was away, I moved in and stripped all of the horrible, dated wallpaper off of the walls in the living room, dining room and kitchen. (I should add here that she had already told me that she planned to do it herself when she came home.)

During that time of working on the house, I fell in love. The house is surrounded on three sides by an old-fashioned porch, which hangs out over the steep lawn and down to the creek and dock. When you sit in the living room, or on the porch, you look out over the creek and to the woods beyond. During my work breaks, I would sit and absorb the peaceful sounds of the water and the birds that congregate in the pear tree just off the porch.

Chauncey Creek is located in Kittery Point, Maine, just over the bridge from Portsmouth, New Hampshire. My mother used to talk about "that feeling" you get when you cross over one of the bridges into Maine. It's a combination of smell, light, and energy. The pace slows. There is the smell of salt and brine. Freshly mowed grass and earth. It's seacoast. It's country. It's a promise of relaxation and introspection.

I've enjoyed many aspects of Kittery Point and the Maine coast on my many trips there, but the corner of the porch is where I spent many vacations. There are times when I need a place to unwind and recharge—my happy place. I saw my daughters and grandchildren. I stayed in my "jammies" until noon. I sipped wine or Margaritas every afternoon while watching the sun fade off the creek and visiting with friends who stopped by.

I watched the inaugural flight of baby house finches, enjoyed the spectacular show of rhododendron, sat in awe as the myriad birds came to the pear tree on their way to somewhere else, and laughed and cried with a special friend who shares this wonderful place with me. I came home rested and refreshed with my "happy place" vision more enhanced.

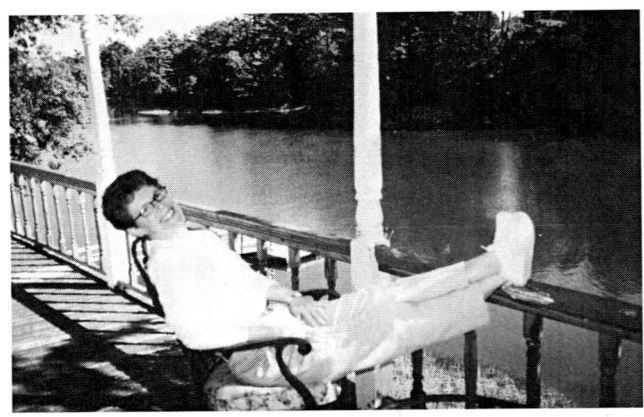

Ellie Gibeau, a great friend.

The Creek

By Ellie Gibeau

The Creek is where you'll find me
on early summer days.
It's where I come for solace
and to reassess and laze.

I sit in my favorite corner
on the porch that sees the Creek.
The water shines and sparkles
and the trees and seagulls speak.

The shadows dance along the shore
and the kingfisher circles his prey.
The tide comes in and then retreats
as it acknowledges another day.

Afternoon brings new reflection
as the birds and shadows dance.
Memories of happy times,
of sadness and happenstance.

Life's journey unfolds before me,
past and future stories told,
As the Creek forges its journey
to the ocean's vast hold.

The Creek becomes our metaphor
for all that life will be,
The ebb and flow of water
and the creation of history.

Thank you for this special place
to reflect and ponder life.
For the time to sit quietly
without the stress and strife.

I look forward to another year,
the seasons come and gone.
To return once more to Mopsy's Creek
where life just flows along.

Katie's Letter

November 2011—Team Mopsy

My mother was diagnosed with Parkinson's disease in 1992 when my brother and I were still in high school. She was 48 years old. For many years I was in denial—and because her symptoms were slow to reveal themselves, I was able to get away with it. I went through two more years of high school and four years of college without telling anyone, even my closest friends. I barely talked about it with my mom and rarely asked her how she was feeling.

But after a while (too long), I realized that my ignoring my mother's disease was not fair to her, or supportive of her. I was in law school in Philadelphia, living six hours from home, so I lacked the ability to physically help her in ways that could have been helpful: I couldn't go to her doctor's appointments with her or run errands, like her friends were able to do. I started thinking that there had to be something I could do, even from afar. In 2004, after doing a little research, I found out about the Parkinson's Unity Walk in New York City. I was drawn to the Unity Walk because of its commitment to finding a cure through re-search, a cause that is near and dear to my mother's heart. The Unity Walk was the perfect way for me to get in-volved, no matter how far from my mother I lived. It was also a wonderful way for me to tell my friends about my mother's fight with the disease and shed light on a sub-ject many of them knew little about. I signed up and invit-ed a few friends to join me. Because my mom lives in Maine, I didn't expect her to make the long trip—but she did, along with a crew of best friends that she has known for years. Team Mopsy (my mother's nickname) was born.

The first year, I sent letters in the mail and e-mails, but had no sense of how much money I might raise. I set Team Mopsy's target at $2,500. We raised almost $10,000. After a few years, Team Mopsy broke into the Top 25 Teams and has remained in the Top 25 for the past five years. In 2011, Team Mopsy had its biggest year yet, raising over $14,000 and being ranked as the 14th highest fundraising team! In all, Team Mopsy has raised over $170,000 since 2004, an amazing accomplishment for a small team relying on individual donations. I am consistently amazed and hum-bled that the same people who supported Team Mopsy eight years ago come back year after year to support our efforts. I am so proud of the money that we have raised for the effort of finding a cure for Parkinson's.

My mom always commends me for my fundraising efforts and tells me how proud she is of me. But what I want her to remember is that the generous donations Team Mopsy receives year after year from friends and family around the country are not because of me—it's all because of her. Team Mopsy's success is a true testament to how beloved my mother is to so many people and to how much we are all proud of her as she bravely lives with this disease—for over twenty years now.

I recently moved from Philadelphia to Boston, in part to live closer to my mom. I was on the board of a great local organization in Philly, The Parkinson Council, and had to resign when I moved. As one of the other board members (who is living with the disease himself) aptly and touchingly put it when I told him I was moving to be closer to my mom, "There is nothing more significant to a Parkinsonian than a devoted daughter." I couldn't have put it better myself.

I love you, Mom. Go Team Mopsy!
Katie Crawford

How Did You Die?

Doc Ann's Favorite*

Did you tackle the trouble that came your way
With a resolute heart and cheerful,
Or hide your face from the light of day
With a craven soul, and fearful?
O, a trouble's a ton or a trouble's an ounce
Or a trouble's what you make it.
It isn't the fact that you're hurt that counts
But only—how did you take it?

You're beaten to earth. Well, well, what's that?
Look up with a smiling face!
It's nothing against you to fall down flat
But—to lie there—that's a disgrace.
The harder you fall, why the higher you bounce.
Be proud of your blackened eye!
It isn't the fact that you're licked that counts—
It's *how* did you fight and *why*.

And, if you be done to the death, what then?

If you battled the best you could,

If you played your part in the world to the end,

Why, the Critic will call it good!

Death comes with a crawl or comes with a pounce,

But whether he's slow or spry,

It isn't the fact that you're dead that counts

But only—how did you die?

*Dr. Ann Tomkins Gibson, founder of Singing Eagle Lodge, 1917

Acknowledgments

This book was written based not on journal writings, but totally on memory, in the form of vignettes written over the past few years, from my experiencing Parkinson's for twenty-eight years now. I can vouch for its basic accurateness. Please forgive me if I have done you wrong. I apologize if I have forgotten anyone.

I give great credit to family members and friends who kept saying, "Write your story. You have a lot to share." Many people made this book possible because they made my life possible.

FAMILY:

• My parents, Elizabeth and Henry Kowal, for hearing me and being such loving supports.

• Susan, my sister, and Jack Rose, her husband, for keeping in touch and helping me out with my early diagnosis.

• My brother Bob Kowal, for pitching in to help Steve, and Pat, my sister-in-law and an author in her own right, for giving me suggestions as I first worked on my book.

• My brother Steve, for scraping me off the floor due to my many falls, for being "Farmer Steve," for cooking many meals and being there. Steve has a flock of grandchildren—twelve actually, ten from one family that includes four who make up the Kowal Family Band. Check them out on YouTube!.

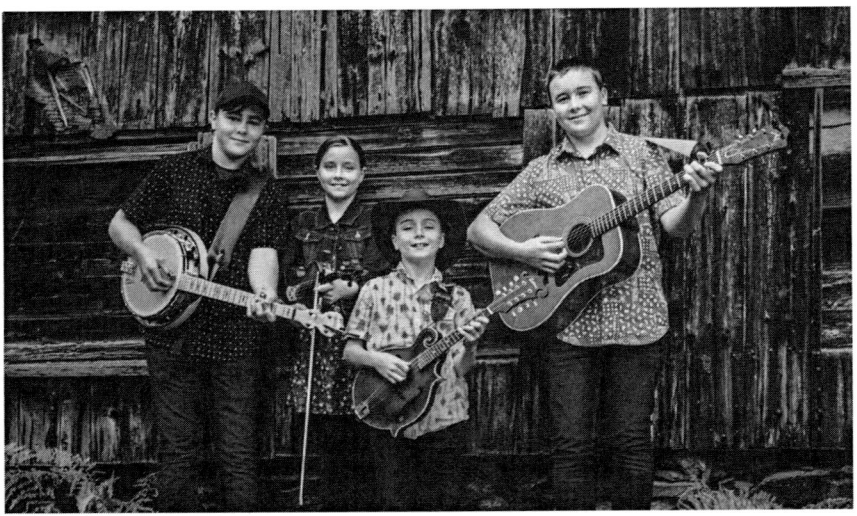

• My daughter Katie for giving me suggestions for my book and putting up with my taking so long in getting my book published. But, my appreciation goes far beyond that. Katie has been a real treasure in my life. She moved to Boston to be closer to me and has been extremely helpful in taking me to doctor appointments, dealing with Extended Family, and helping me to make my life easier. She's always on top of things. I value all that she does for me. What a daughter!

• My son Stephen I value and treasure greatly. He has often gone the extra mile for me. Christmas 2019 when I was in very poor shape, worse than today, he, along with

Katie and Arabella, made it possible for me to visit them in Baltimore. Stephen escorted me on both my flights, flying back and forth two round trips from Manchester, NH to Baltimore, MD. When Extended Family a year ago couldn't arrange coverage for me, rather than risk my being alone, in spite of his work schedule, Stephen came to help me out. What a son!

• Arabella has been a wonderful addition in my life. She goes out of her way to show me things I need to do or know. She insisted on taking me to the Social Security office to make sure I was receiving all the benefits I was entitled to. It was worth the trip. She's also been a marvelous resource for trouble shooting my computer problems. Stephen and Arabella have blessed me with very special grandchildren who give me much joy.

• Alex, Luke and Anna, my incredible grandchildren, who are bright, spirited and loving. They help their "Gami" deal with Parkinson's, picking up things I've dropped and getting me things I need. They love pushing me in my wheelchair. I appreciate them being inquisitive about why I can't do certain things such as standing up from a chair. It feels good answering their questions.

• My aunt Peggy Howe, for encouraging me and having wonderful conversations by phone.

- Don Goodrich, who after Sally's death, continues to have a part in the Peter M. Goodrich Foundation.

- Mark Donavon, Sally's brother, for stopping to visit on his way up into Maine.

- My cousin Jim Averill and his wife Janet, for their constant and generous support for the Parkinson's Unity Walk.

- Mary Hill, a special cousin, and Carlos, for visiting me and introducing me to Alexa.

- My brother-in-law David Crawford and his wife Beth, for continuing to include me in the Crawford family.

- My sister-in-law and friend Linda Hansen Rodier, for continuing our wonderful friendship.

WRITERS GROUP:

- I greatly appreciate the genuine loving and trusting support of my writers' group: Mary Jane Rowan, Susan DeVito, Lynda True, Glenny Dunbar and leader Rebecca Dawson-Webb, a remarkably kind woman who offers validation that is very real. Also thanks to Elizabeth Kirschner, leader of the first writers' group I joined, as well as fellow writer Dwyer Vessey.

CHURCH COMMUNITY:

- First Congregational Church of Kittery at Kittery Point, Pastor Brian Gruhn and his wife Emily; Jeff Gallager, former pastor and role model for writing a book, and Jack Lynes and his wife Kris, Maren C. Tirabassi and Linda Hurst, who all served as interim ministers.

• A.M. McCurdy, for giving me encouragement and honest feedback, and for driving me to Marcia Gibbons' so I could read rough drafts of the vignettes to her before she died; A.M.'s husband, Garvin, and their daughter Morgan for all their help, support and kindnesses. Also, Sarah (Marcia Gibbons' daughter) and Peter Drummond for keeping in touch, checking on me and bringing me goodies.

• Sara Rhoades, who helped with organizing the vignettes. Mary and Jon Carter for initiating the Parkinson's Walk in Kittery. Leslie Culbert, a bright spirit who calls me Sunshine. Linda Browning, mortgage broker for both Bridgit and me who approved our mortgage loans for our homes on Chauncey Creek.

• Sybil Becker and Bonnie Frisbee. Gail and Rick Leonard, and Maureen Bilodeau who helped me out at the beginning; Sally Sulloway, Laurie Smith, Lynn and Chuck Hatch, Paula and Dave Bradstreet, Ellie and Charlie Kirkpatrick. Tim and Carolyn Roy, Diane Harvey, Steve and Geneve Hoffman, Mark Lechner, Amy Richards, Linda Powell, Beth St. John, Traci Pardue who helped me set up my PayPal account; Jennifer Gray, Della O'Shea, Jan and Brian Redonets, Mel and Donna Stobbs, Gudrun Carver, Candace

DeLisio, Sue Brown, Merry and Don Craig, Gail and Tony Barrington, Sheelah Pearson, and oh, so many others.

• Also, Charlotte Small, who through Lotsa Helping Hands coordinated my calendar of appointments to schedule rides each week with people who had volunteered to help take me places. She was a wonderful help to me. Her commitment was remarkable and I personally thank her.

KITTERY COMMUNITY:

• Elisa Kiernan, who has been cleaning for me since I've lived in Kittery, and her husband Mark, the miracle man who can figure out how to fix anything that needs fixing; they have so gone out of their way to help me. Kathy Connor, master gardener who remarkably has volunteered to take care of my garden for fourteen years. My foot massager Bridgit Holzer and her husband Rich, two good friends down the road; and Galen Beale, for stopping in frequently and keeping me up to date on Kittery goings-on. Camille and Matt Brady, always responsive and helpful; they've been good friends since our Mass Mutual days. He traded in his computer for a hammer and now does carpentry and renovation work. Martha Peterson, Debby Ronnquist, Sally Hirschberg, Heather Thomsen and her late husband Len, who had Parkinson's and who listened to some of these vignettes. Also, Dianne Dean, Ann Grinnell, Marge Pelletier. Pat and Vaughn Kailian, Pat DeGrandpre, Wendy Turner and Paula Ickeringill.

SINGING EAGLE LODGE:

• My long-time friends from Singing Eagle Lodge, Susan Kemp, Linda Briggs; Judy Hunter, and her sisters Jill and Jan; Lynn Luzzi, Laura Livingston, Amy Shorey, Peach Parke, Candy Alcauskas and Anne ("Pickle") Knight. These friends have been my lifelong supporters and I am grateful for their ongoing love.

ST. AGNES (these are all original names):

• Wynne Edwards, Chris Evans, Nancy Fenster, Joyce Hamm, Tessa Miller (Melvin), Alexandra Northrop, Carol Nostrand, Helen Pittinger, Linda Shincel, Corki VanKleeck, Holly Wilson and Gail Thalmann.

SKIDMORE COLLEGE:

• Mary Avery, Nancy Nevell, Melinda and Sky Bridgman, Marguerite Borrie, Bonnie Rosenthal, Susan Kanowith and Jill Schuker.

SWEDISH "FAMILY":

• Sister and brother Lena and Lars Helgstrand, and Johan, their younger brother who was four years old at the time, and their parents Annie and Rolf Lindh, with whom I spent the summer of '64 in Enköping, Sweden. I got to make many friends like Per Eckerborn, a Swedish participant, and others as part of the Experiment in International Living, a program that dates back to 1932.

OTHER FRIENDS:

• Ellie Gibeau, Bennett Swingle, Nancy Thayer, Nancy Stoer, Marcia Vose, Carol Chapuis, Ed Mullen, Dorean Kimball, Fran Philippe, Kathe and David Chipman, Pam Marble, Charlie Simpson, and Larry Kristopher, who could cut my hair with his eyes closed—he cut it for 17 years.

BOOK RELATED:

• As mentioned in the introduction, Tessa Melvin, Liz Korabek-Emerson and Nancy Grossman, and my daughter Katie.

MEDICAL RELATED:

• Michael Kleinman, MD, Neurologist; Trevor Braden, MD, PCP; Jerry Parrota, my outpatient physical therapist from York Hospital and Tina Trivino, my massage therapist. Also, Cathi Thomas from the Boston University Medical Center.

NORTHEAST REHAB:

• Sarah Conant and Carol Bullen, and everyone there, as well as Lisa Sommers who was there from the start, but who's moved on. PTs Julie Bastille and Dave Lashure, OT Laurie Lavoie and speech pathologist Terri Walsh.

EXTENDED FAMILY:

• Mary Spaulding, Emma Lynch-Callaghan (my soul mate),

Jeannie Rudman, Connie Bruni, Sandy Camire, Jennifer Stillings and Maria Jebari. After a year of 24/7 care, I've come to appreciate the value of caretakers—once I got over the hurdle of accepting help while trading off privacy and independence.

About the Author

Martha has been a mother, daughter, sister, grandmother, friend, camper and councillor, tennis player, all-round athlete, gypsy and pilot. She earned her Bachelors degree from Skidmore College in 1966, and her Master's degree in Counseling and Student Personnel Services from Purdue University in 1973, the same month she became a pilot.

She always knew she could earn a Master's degree, but learning to fly took her out of her comfort zone, something that Parkinson's disease would also do. She has dealt with this condition for twenty-eight years with grace, courage, and determination.